WHY DOESN'T MY DOCTOR KNOW THIS?

Conquering Irritable Bowel Syndrome, Inflammatory Bowel Disease, Crohn's Disease and Colitis

constipation

ulcers

blood

pain gas

indigestion

spasms

heartburn

bloating

diarrhea reflux

GERD

DAVID DAHLMAN, DC

Foreword by Jeffrey Bland, Ph.D., FACN

madeeasy
PUBLISHING

AN IMPRINT OF MORGAN JAMES PUBLISHING

WHY DOESN'T MY DOCTOR KNOW THIS?

By David Dahlman, DC
© 2008 All rights reserved.

ISBN: 978-1-60037-316-9 (Paperback)

Library of Congress Control Number: 2007935675

Published by:

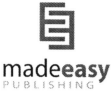

AN IMPRINT OF MORGAN JAMES PUBLISHING

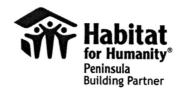

Morgan James Publishing, LLC
1225 Franklin Ave. Suite 325
Garden City, NY 11530-1693
800.485.4943
www.MorganJamesPublishing.com

Cover & Interior Designs by:

Megan Johnson
Johnson2Design
www.Johnson2Design.com
megan@Johnson2Design.com

DISCLAIMER

The information and advice in this book are based on the training, personal and professional experiences and research of the author. Its contents are current and accurate; however, the information presented is not intended to substitute for professional medical advice. The author and publisher urge you to consult with your physician or other qualified health-care provider prior to starting any treatment or undergoing any surgical procedure. Because there is always some risk involved, the author and publisher cannot be responsible for any adverse effects or consequences resulting from the use of any of the suggestions, preparations, supplements or procedures described in this book.

WHY DOESN'T MY DOCTOR KNOW THIS?

Conquering Irritable Bowel Syndrome, Inflammatory Bowel Disease, Crohn's Disease, and Colitis

WHAT OTHERS SAY

Your program has CURED my ulcerative colitis. I said CURED. Prior to beginning your program I had diarrhea that evolved slowly over a period of years from a few times a day to up to 15 times daily for close to a year. I had tried Pepto Bismol, Lomotil, Imodium AD, and then traditional doctor's prescriptions, each of which worked somewhat initially, but then failed. I went to gastrointestinal specialists, did the colonoscopy thing, including removal of a polyp. Nothing worked . I was desperate as my life revolved around the toilet, and left me weak and tired. I searched the internet for answers.

I ran across your program on an internet search. I read your material that seemed to make sense, and decided to try it. Within a couple of WEEKS of the strict diet and faithfully taking the recommended supplements, my diarrhea was gone. (After YEARS of suffering.)

Taking your emailed advice, I continued on the entire program for three months, remaining diarrhea-free. I began eating a limited amount of gluten without a problem. After about 3 months of "normal" bowel movements I decided that prior to adding other foods on the restricted list, I would try going off the supplements to try to eliminate and isolate the possibility that the types of foods could only be eaten if the supplements were continued. I continued on the supplement-free with some gluten scenario for about a month, and then began ingesting small amounts of dairy, such as in the label ingredients on some prepared foods.

I was still symptom-free, so after about another month, I began eating all foods except peanuts, again with no problems. It is now about 8 months since I began the program, a good 6 months since my diarrhea stopped, 4 months since I stopped taking the supplements, and three months since I began a normal diet. I now eat whatever I want, including peanuts, and am COMPLETELY CURED of the ulcerative colitis. I gave my internist doctor a copy of your program. I don't know what use he has made of it, since I haven't seen him for some time now.

Ron S.

WHY DOESN'T MY DOCTOR KNOW THIS?

Conquering Irritable Bowel Syndrome, Inflammatory Bowel Disease, Crohn's Disease, and Colitis

Dear Dr. Dahlman,

I don't know how to thank you for your commitment to making a difference in people's lives. Your research and program and how you're put everything together has changed my life in a week. I have never been able to eat solid food more than once a day and couldn't go to the bathroom even with once a day without using an aloe vera laxative.

It has been one week since I've followed everything you've told me to do and the swelling and pain is gone and today for the first time in years, I had a normal, solid bowel movement without any pain. I am able to eat a little bit at breakfast and lunch along with the supplements you prescribed and I can see that I am beginning to tolerate them better each day.

I have called everyone I know that either treats patients with colitis and Crohn's or people who are currently on medication for this. I am referring everyone I know to you, including people who have arthritis because your report is so thorough, it's like a roadmap from the beginning of the problem to where we have all wound up.

They say each one of us should leave the world in a better place than we found it, I can certainly say that you have definitely done that by helping me and so many others. You are really making a difference in the world, God bless you Dr. Dahlman.

Sincerely,

Jan

in New York

Just a note for your files:

2 years ago I read your IBS protocol because true to form I had tried a heck of a lot of things to help myself...........I was advanced with holistic modalities but was becoming unable to travel even by car because of the unpredictable GI problems.....

I am now 90% predictable and that is good enough for me to travel again.......I was able to do this with your outline.............I am an O blood type so simply eliminating DAIRY 100% and taking various supplements at the beginning of the protocol put me in good steed.

Because I DID NOT follow your outline to a T it took me 1 year to get here.........I KNOW that had I done what you said exactly I would have had complete resolution in just a few months......

I have gained 25lbs. That is a mixed blessing I suppose. However when I was younger, all I ever wanted to do was not LOOSE an ounce and I was usually scared that If I ate the wrong thing I would loose a few pounds by the next day and for an IBS kid that was FRIGHTNING!! WE know what that feels like and WE know what that means!!!!!!!!!! No one else does.

Sincerely,

Trish F.

Pickerington Ohio

✳   ✳   ✳   ✳

*H*ello Dr. Dahlman,

I just wanted to thank you and all of your hard work on your research. Your diet has turned my life around. I can go out and not worry about having to find a bathroom or have constant pain in my side anymore. I still refer back to your information and am glad it is there.

Thank you,

Melanie

✳   ✳   ✳   ✳

Hi Dr Dahlman,

I just thought you'd like to know I followed your suggestions and everything is back to normal. My doctor had already set me up for colonoscopy, barium enema, etc, etc, etc! I told him forget it I'll take care of it myself. I know he thinks I'm crazy but only time will tell who's right and who's wrong!

Thank you again for allowing people access to helping themselves. God bless you.

Shirley

Dr D:

Were it not for your guidance and step-by-step program, I would have ended up on disability. I am typing this from my desk at work. I recommend taking the consultations in addition to the nutritional therapies. That's what worked for me, and I was just about hopeless.

You can use my name.

Deborah P.

Dr. Dahlman,

Just a quick note to let you know I'm still doing VERY WELL!!! This is just wonderful, to be able to live a normal life again is so exciting. Your treatment is the only thing that worked, and the fact that you took time with me to actually figure out the problem was unbelievable. My gastro said these words, "Don't eat a lot of fat". That was it, my entire solution, according to him was to not eat a lot of fat. I've had problems now for decades, this is like a miracle. My heartfelt thanks go out to you.

Thanks so much,

Karin

✳   ✳   ✳   ✳

Dr. Dahlman,

Just wanted to say thanks for the great website and all your help. I don't know if you remember us talking but after a flu shot I had diarrhea for almost 7 weeks. I went to my Dr. and a gastro. ----right!!! After seven days on your plan my gut turned around. You don't know how much I appreciate your help.

Thanks again,

Dave H.

✳   ✳   ✳   ✳

Dr Dahlman,

I just want to let you know that I am still symptom-free after several months of being off the supplements. I still take food enzymes occasionally, but I am not experiencing the gas and IBS symptoms at all. I am so grateful to you and your program. I am back to eating most of the foods that I had to let go of while on the program. There's not much I can't eat. I haven't tried tofu yet and eat few beans, but that's OK.

Thank you so much for sharing this with all of us. What a gift! I was skeptical and didn't have much hope when we started working together. Then when I didn't see the success I expected after the three months, I was really discouraged. But, after doing the intense dose of the Ultra Clear Sustain, things drastically improved.

Take care and keep up the good work. I tell everyone I know about your program in hopes that they will take advantage of it. I'm happy to share my story of recovery from IBS. I NEVER thought I'd be free of it.

Thanks again,

Nanci Z

*D*r. D,

Just a byte to express my appreciation for your IBS program. I have to admit I'm a well-schooled skeptic. I never expected those annoying and agonizing symptoms to shrink to mere shadows. My wife says she can now take me out in public without fear of embarrassment. I am grateful. She is ecstatic.

I even dared to share the news with my family doctor. As soon as I uttered the word wellness, his eyes glazed over as he doodled aimlessly across his Rx pad. I have to give him some credit. He didn't pass judgment, he didn't scoff. He just said, "I recommend you have a colonoscopy." His voice was neutral but his eyes had a sort of punitive glint.

So I traipsed off to my favorite gastroenterologist. Of course he had to ask if I was taking anything for my irritable bowel. It's required by the HMO handbook. I started to tell him about the diet and the supplements. At first he smiled patronizingly. You know that look. It's the same one you got when you told your mother about the monster under your bed. Then I noticed he wasn't there anymore. I know I can be boring but really.

Then the nurse whispered conspiratorially into my ear, "What's his name?"

She was so sincere I started to spell it our for her, "D-A-L-H, no, it's D-E-H-L, no, no, it's D-A-H-L-M..." I felt a little twitch in my arm as the sedative pulsed through the IV. The rest is a blank.

Thank you, thank you, thank you. Without your program I couldn't even contemplate traveling to Italy to visit the grandchildren this year or maybe ever.

Jim U.

*D*ear Dr. Dahlman,

I would like to thank you for all you have done to help me with my IBS. It has been well over 5 months since beginning your program, and I am happy to report that I am feeling fantastic! I have added dairy back into my diet, as well as some of my favorite spicy foods and still so far so good. The hardest part is getting used to the idea that I can eat whatever I want, I guess the fear is still there that something will set if off again. Slowly I am beginning to believe that my IBS may be gone for good.

Thanks to you and your generosity I am living a much happier life!

Sincerely,

Leeanne

Dear Dr. Dahlman,

I just wanted to take a moment and say "Thank You". I ended my formal treatment for IBS with you the beginning of February. While I was undergoing treatment, there were some major changes for the better that happened. Since my treatment has ended, I still continue to see these wonderful changes that have given me my life back. I am at the point now where I can eat anything I want and I no longer live in fear. I am no longer anxious about what will bring on an attack, which at the height of my IBS it was just about everything. I am the calm, level - headed person I used to be. I am enjoying life again, only more because I appreciate it. My husband thanks you as well for giving him his wife back. I am much healthier and feel so much better. I recommend you whenever I can. You are a lifesaver!

Thank You again for all you do.

Sincerely,

Elise H.

* * * *

Dr. Dahlman,

I am feeling, eating and pooping great! You definitely know what you are doing, and I cannot thank you enough!

George

* * * *

WHAT OTHERS SAY

$\mathcal{D}$r. Dahlman,

Just thought you might appreciate my posting of this to the IBS Group bulletin board:

Hi all, and have not posted much but have a lot to say on the subject. I have been struggling with IBS C for almost 30 years (I am 45 now). I have spent over $50,000 in my search for answers, seeing doctors, therapists, hypnotists, new age specialists, psychics, acupuncturists etc., and experimenting with every product and approach under the sun to help my body get well. Everything was a quick fix. I was like a junkie trying to find a new hit. I had originally concluded that I would just be addicted to laxatives and colonics to clean my system out and avoid the pain etc. and just accept that my body was screwed up forever. I know the agony that many of you go through day to day. Believe me I do.

In the last few months, after being a patient of Dr. David Dahlman, my constipation does not exist. He has worked independently with me to tailor a program (diet and supplements) that meets my unique situation. The big change for me was saying goodbye to ALL dairy. Being the nacho queen that I am, this was not easy at all until I started feeling the payoff of his plan. Over the years, I had so many colonics and relied heavily on laxatives, my body forgot how to work on its own. Progress was slow initially, I was like a junkie going clean but I must say life is looking absolutely wonderful right now. Lazarus has risen. I have now dropped 30 pounds and I am off antidepressants. My self-assessment of my health of my body on a scale of 1 to 10 was a 1 in January of this year. It is now a 6+. I am still working on killing some bad bacteria that are residing in me and causing some issues, but I am well on my way to being free of the prison I have been in for so many years. Believe me, I am grateful and am now experiencing freedom.

Carol G.

✳   ✳   ✳   ✳

$\mathcal{D}$ear Dr. Dahlman,

I don't think I have ever written a thank-you note to a doctor in my life! However, you are no ordinary doctor and, as such, are deserving of just that. Doctor, I need to simply say thank you for giving my life back to me! I still cannot believe the "miracle" you worked on me. Words cannot explain how horrible my life was before I came to you; the pain was extreme and never-ending. But now? Now, I am free of the pain! I feel WONDERFUL! You have simply given my life back to me and for that I will be forever grateful. I stand in total awe of your knowledge and expertise! I thank you from the bottom of my heart!

Karen W.

ACKNOWLEDGEMENTS

First, I'll thank my father. At first glance, it might seem a bit silly…everyone should thank their Dad. Gift of life, guidance, discipline and support, a couple extra bucks here and there. But I go back to that day my senior year in high school, a couple months from graduation, when I left track practice and was headed to the locker room. Uncle Charlie was there to pick me up. That was odd. He said hurry, he'll explain in a minute.

I'm sure you can imagine what his explanation was. But that day, as bad as the news was and unbeknownst to me at the time, was the catalyst and true reason I am doing what I'm doing today.

Dad's death, I believe at first subconsciously and not consciously till I was in my early 20's, made me ultimately question conventional medicine and decide it just made sense that my health and longevity would be greatly enhanced if I watched my diet and learned as much as possible about nutrition, herbs, vitamins, minerals, and other "alternative" therapies. This was back in the 1970's, we've come a long way. Thanks Dad!

My semi-formal education about alternative health came from a couple places before my formal chiropractic and nutrition degrees. I must thank the late David Polen, DC who took me under his wing for a year and allowed me to watch his thinking and cutting edge treatments…sometimes a bit too cutting edge for his own good. What I learned from him was a post graduate degree in itself.

A colleague of his, James LaValle, R.Ph., C.C.N., N.D. deserves even more thanks as, at first my doctor who helped me enhance my health, then as a friend who was amazingly supportive of my decision to become a chiropractor and open an alternative health clinic that he knew would ultimately compete with his. I appreciate his vast knowledge about everything "alternative" and his willingness to share it. I also appreciate lessons learned about men and our egos and how they get in the way. I am forever in his debt.

Dr. Paul Goldberg, DC one of my nutrition professors, was in the room and because of him…though unbeknownst to him…when a light bulb went off in my head and I realized the importance of the gastrointestinal system in maintaining human health and that its imbalances may be the cause of many health conditions.

How could I not thank Cristi Maue Kessler for starting me on the path of visiting health foods stores and teaching me how to prepare real and healthy meals. And, my son Ian, as a little boy putting up with my lengthy and incessant conversations with people I didn't know at health food stores as I learned to speak the language of health. He finally learned to ask me not to talk to anyone as we walked into the store.

My editor, Elaine Sparber also deserves a thanks, especially for putting up with my own self caused delays and for taking a rough manuscript and putting order to it.

FOREWORD

What constitutes a health book worth reading? In my experience of 35 years in the field it comes down to information that can be applied in people's lives that makes a difference in their health. I have had a number of unsolicited conversations with people who have had various intestinal problems including irritable bowel syndrome and inflammatory bowel disorders who have found Dr. Dahlman's information and program that he describes in his book *"Why Doesn't My Doctor Know This? Conquering Irritable Bowel Syndrome, Inflammatory Bowel Disease, Crohn's Disease and Colitis"* and have had tremendous success with the program.

We all know that no solution works for all people, but when I hear of people who for years have been plagued with digestive problems that have had their issues resolved by applying the concepts described in Dr. Dahlman's book I listen carefully. Although Dr. Dahlman is not a gastroenterologist, he is a health professional that has focused his interest on nutrition and its relationship to health.

Through his studies and insight he has developed the program described in his book that seems to provide many people the resolution to their problem that they have been searching for. I think that his program is sensible and can be applied easily by anyone searching for a way to improve their digestive function. It is based upon both basic science and clinical research that represents the cutting edge of our understanding of the cause of many of the cases of digestive disorders.

I recommend this book for anyone who would like to explore a new approach to managing complex digestive problems through the use of diet and nutritional therapy.

Jeffrey Bland, PhD, FACN

WHY DOESN'T MY DOCTOR KNOW THIS?

Conquering Irritable Bowel Syndrome, Inflammatory Bowel Disease, Crohn's Disease, and Colitis

CONTENTS

WHY DOESN'T MY DOCTOR KNOW THIS?

Conquering Irritable Bowel Syndrome, Inflammatory Bowel Disease, Crohn's Disease, and Colitis

INTRODUCTION

When I think of irritable bowel syndrome (IBS), I think not only of my patients, but also of myself. And my memories of my battle with the disorder are not good. (Are anyone's?) I still vividly remember the days interrupted by the search for a bathroom, the pain, the discomfort, the embarrassment, and the loss of quality of life.

My personal battle with IBS started while I was sitting in a plastic chair on the deck of a restaurant talking with a friend. I found that I had rubbed some skin off my elbow on the arm of the chair. I thought nothing of it until a couple of days later when, within the span of a couple of hours, my elbow swelled to the size of a golf ball. The diagnosis: staph infection.

Considering the amount of the swelling and the pain and the heat associated with it, and upon the advice of a conventional medical doctor, I decided to take an antibiotic. My elbow hurt, the swelling and the pain were hampering my activities, and I believed I knew enough about what I was doing that I could probably mediate any damage the antibiotics might cause to my gastrointestinal system.

A few weeks after I completed the course of antibiotics, my gastrointestinal problems began. They started with some gurgling noises, which quickly turned to diarrhea. I also had stomachaches and lots of gas and bloating. I had to go four or five times a day, and brother, when I had to go, you had better get out of my way. I can still remember how frustrated I felt the morning I tried to leave my hotel in Chicago to run the Chicago Marathon but had to turn my car around in the parking lot so I could hightail it back up to my room and use the bathroom just one more time before hitting the starting line. IBS was quickly changing my life.

So being the really great doctor I was sure I was, I put myself on the treatment plan I was using with my patients at the time. Knowing full well the antibiotics had probably altered or damaged my beneficial bacteria population, which is so necessary for gastrointestinal health, my game plan was to take the same product I recommended to my patients for the reestablishment of this population.

The most common species of beneficial bacteria are *Lactobacillus acidophilus* and *Bifidobacterium*. These are also known as probiotics, the opposite of antibiotics. I always told my patients, "If you ever have to take an antibiotic, also take a probiotic while you're on the antibiotic and for one to two months afterward." I wasn't exactly the best patient because

I didn't begin taking the probiotic as soon as I should have. And I paid for it. This personal experience reinforced what I always suspected: It doesn't take large doses of antibiotics to alter the proper balance of beneficial bacteria and set into motion the cascade of events that leads to symptoms.

The plan in this book is as effective and complete as it is due to what I learned through my own experience. Time kept passing and I couldn't seem to shake my problem. I began to wonder what kind of a doctor I was if I couldn't fix myself. I therefore began to research additional natural products, the significance of bacteria levels, and how to interpret lab results in different ways. It took some time and patience, but the end result was that I figured it out and sent my IBS packing in less than three months.

Relief from IBS cannot be found by taking a pill. The same way that a headache is not caused by a lack of Tylenol floating around in the bloodstream, IBS is not caused by a lack of whatever medication the pharmaceutical industry is currently pushing. This means that the conventional medical world does not and never will have a cure for IBS, only medications to suppress its individual symptoms. Which means that no one pill will ever solve the mystery called IBS. Which means that it's up to you to find the solution to your own problem. And there is a solution.

The first step in the process is understanding that IBS—as well as all gastrointestinal conditions, including Crohn's Disease and any type of colitis—is a complex problem requiring a complex solution. I have identified nine distinct variables that combine to cause the symptoms of IBS or any other gastrointestinal condition, and have developed a comprehensive plan to reverse or repair their ill effects. My plan is the end product of my many years of treating thousands of people with IBS, and I have learned how to explain it in an easy-to-understand manner.

This book began as an educational pamphlet I handed out in my office and then grew into a longer booklet I made available on my website. Its title comes from my patients. "Why doesn't my doctor know this?" is the question I'm most frequently asked by the patients in my office.

My patients are right. Why don't most doctors know the causes of IBS and how to treat the disorder? This lack of knowledge is among the biggest failures of conventional medicine, and we'll discuss it later in the book.

For those of you suffering from inflammatory bowel disease (IBD), such as Crohn's disease or any form of colitis, understanding the information about IBS that I present in this book is very important. Your IBD probably began as a case of IBS and then progressed to a more complex and severe condition. The successful treatment of your IBD will build upon the information about IBS that I present here, with the couple of changes I describe in Chapter 9, "Crohn's Disease and Any Type of Colitis." Reading the entire book in a step-by-step manner will help you apply the advice in Chapter 9.

Prior to my personal experience with IBS, I was able to help many, but not all, of my patients get better. Now, because of the refinements I've made to my plan, the vast majority of my patients see a complete elimination of any uncomfortable symptoms associated with their gastrointestinal tracts in an average of three months.

If you've been dealing with IBS for a while, you may have read some other books available on the disorder. These books seem to fall into four categories: those that suggest diet is completely at fault, with a large number of pages devoted to recipes (if it were that easy, no one would have IBS!); those that suggest diet, stress, and psychological issues are the cause (let's blame the patient!) with the book focusing on lifestyle modifications; those that offer great information but no plan for recovery; and those whose authors seem to want to impress you with how much they know about the subject, instead of telling you only and exactly what you need to feel better. None of these books discusses antibiotics and their effect on beneficial bacteria levels and subsequent effects on the gastrointestinal tract. And most importantly, none of the available books offers a step-by-step treatment plan.

The solution to IBS is actually very simple. And I do know how silly that may sound to someone who has been suffering with the condition, whether for many years or just a short period of time. You haven't been able to find any relief even though you think you've tried everything and you may have been told by your conventional medical doctor either that you must learn to live with your problem or that it's in your head. The reason conventional medical doctors believe this is that they have only one tool at their disposal. This tool is drugs. Drugs only suppress or manage IBS symptoms; they don't offer a cure. We will work to eliminate the causes of your symptoms, and that's why we will succeed.

The premise from which I work is quite simple. There are only two areas of concern when it comes to overcoming the uncomfortable symptoms associated with the gastrointestinal system. These two areas govern the health of the entire gastrointestinal system. They are bacteria and chemistry. Everything that occurs in the gastrointestinal system (the definition of which, for the purpose of our efforts, is that it extends from the lips all the way to the anus) falls into one of these two categories.

If the necessary population of good bacteria that lives inside the gut is altered or damaged, a change in chemistry will eventually take place, in time followed by the beginning of symptoms. Everybody experiences a unique set of symptoms, and the timing of the onset of these symptoms also varies. Some people develop symptoms as children, while others may be in their nineties. IBS does not discriminate because of age.

The primary culprit in the alteration or damage to the population of beneficial bacteria in the gut is antibiotics. Antibiotics are designed to kill bacteria. Normally used to cure infections, they alter a portion of the good bacteria living in the gastrointestinal system as well as killing the bad bacteria. It doesn't matter whether you've taken two or two hundred courses of antibiotics in your lifetime. It also doesn't matter whether you took them only until you were ten years old, have taken them throughout your lifetime, or haven't taken any in the last decade. Each time you took them, you altered or damaged your population of beneficial bacteria, and even though these bacteria are living, reproducing organisms, they don't always reproduce back to proper, balanced levels. Secondary culprits are lack of digestive enzyme, over-the-counter medications, abnormal bacteria, yeast or parasites, prescription medications, and poor diet (including alcohol). All can have detrimental effects on the delicate balance between the good and bad bacteria in the gastrointestinal tract. We all use these products or eat poorly at some time in our lives, don't we?

The good news is that we can quite easily reestablish proper bacterial balance by taking a probiotic. We will also help the chemistry return to normal by feeding the tissue of the gastrointestinal system nutritional supplements with specific healing nutrients.

We will help improve digestion by taking digestive enzymes, which will assure full-strength enzyme activity for the complete breakdown of foods, helping to eliminate gas, bloating, indigestion, heartburn, and reflux (the backflow of a small amount of food from the stomach to the esophagus). These enzymes will also change the pH, or acid-alkaline balance, of the food moving through the system. Once again, a change in chemistry. We will couple this protocol of all-natural products with temporary dietary changes. Of course, any dietary change will cause, in effect, a change in chemistry.

Rounding out the program, for the small percentage of people who might need it, will be laboratory testing, including stool testing for parasites, bacteria, and yeast, and blood testing for food allergies.

From this book, you won't get technical jargon or sleep-inducing explanations of the biochemistry of the body (although you may need some sleep). You also won't be told that your problem is all in your head. It's not, and I know that. If your doctor has told you that you're stressed and made you feel that your condition is your fault, ignore him or her. If those words

INTRODUCTION

were accompanied by a prescription for an antidepressant, realize that what your doctor is really saying is he or she doesn't know what to do for you, so please go home and feel better about feeling so bad.

What you will get from this book is a proven treatment plan for IBS. Chapter 1 explains what IBS is, as well as what it isn't, since the misconceptions abound. Chapter 2 discusses why most conventional medical doctors don't know the information presented in this book, and describes the path, from doctor to doctor and test to test, that you may have traveled as a result. Chapter 3 details the lifestyle influences that can unbalance your gastrointestinal tract and lead to IBS. Chapter 4 begins describing the treatment plan, starting with the supplements that I've found to be invaluable in healing IBS. Chapter 5 presents the Big Four Don't-You-*Dare*-Break-'Em Dietary Rules (stupid name, but there's a reason), and Chapter 6 describes the step-by-step thought process that I use in my office and that will help you as you work your way through my program. Chapter 7 explains why the average person with IBS also has other health complaints. Chapter 8 discusses how to adapt the basic treatment plan for children and teens with IBS, and Chapter 9 describes how to adjust the plan for Crohn's disease and any type of colitis. Chapter 10 reviews hiatal hernia and offers a self-massage technique that aids in its elimination. The books ends with an appendix that reviews some alternative treatments I suggest avoiding and a resource list of supplements and their suppliers for people who have trouble finding suitable supplements locally as well as a discussion of the laboratory tests that some of you will find useful.

Something that this book will not teach you is how to cope with IBS. It will not teach you how to live with the condition, or how to manage it, or how to deal with occasional "flares." It will teach you how to conquer IBS, as well as Crohn's disease and any type of colitis, and become symptom-free, because it will give you a plan. So, let's get started.

WHY DOESN'T MY DOCTOR KNOW THIS?

Conquering Irritable Bowel Syndrome, Inflammatory Bowel Disease, Crohn's Disease, and Colitis

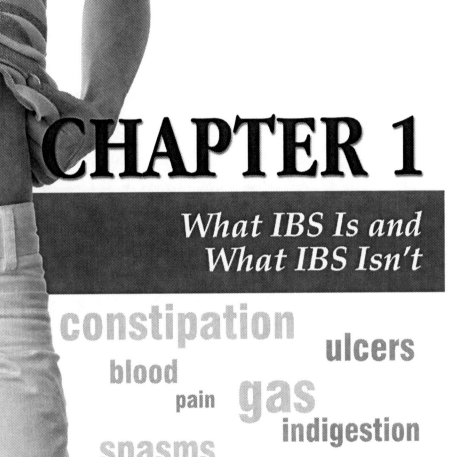

CHAPTER 1

What IBS Is and What IBS Isn't

constipation

blood

pain

ulcers

gas

indigestion

spasms

heartburn

bloating

diarrhea

reflux

GERD

WHY DOESN'T MY DOCTOR KNOW THIS?

Conquering Irritable Bowel Syndrome, Inflammatory Bowel Disease, Crohn's Disease, and Colitis

Discussing what irritable bowel syndrome (IBS) isn't can be just as interesting as discussing what it is. In fact, it might help you more completely understand what IBS is.

If you haven't been able to get an answer to your problem from your conventional medical doctor and you've been trying to figure it out yourself, you may have jumped to a wrong conclusion or two. One common conclusion is that IBS is caused by stress. Since IBS is so prevalent and other family members seem to also have it, another common conclusion is that it's genetic. Much confusion surrounds IBS. In this chapter, we will wash away the misconceptions and define what IBS really is, allowing you to focus on the steps necessary to eliminate your symptoms.

WHAT IBS ISN'T

The researchers who study IBS spend most of their time looking at sophisticated elements of gastrointestinal function and the accompanying laboratory findings. Needless to say, if your gastrointestinal system is unhealthy, you will have many abnormal findings and imbalanced chemical markers. Since most of the research into IBS is sponsored by pharmaceutical companies, the goal of the research is to determine what is out of balance and then to apply and test the medications developed by the sponsoring companies to manage the imbalances. The goal is not to eliminate these imbalances, but just to control them.

Stress and Abnormal Laboratory Findings

Remember the popular philosophical question, "What came first—the chicken or the egg?" Interestingly enough, we can ask that same question about IBS, stress, and functional changes.

Stress

Your stress is not what came first. I can say that with complete certainty. Yes, I know that when you become stressed, your symptoms increase, sometimes reaching the point where they feel like they're out of control. Because of this, it seems to make sense that stress is what's causing your problem. Wrong! Stop thinking like a conventional medical doctor.

It's that failed critical-thought process that has some conventional medical doctors putting people with IBS on antidepressants. The antidepressants will calm these people, whom these doctors believe are always stressed, take life too hard, or are just too emotional about things. The antidepressants may or may not help the IBS. Sometimes they help it for a while, but then the symptoms return. So now these people with IBS symptoms are also on medications that produce their own side effects, with no plan to get off them.

What we're faced with here is the age-old chicken-or-egg question. What came first—the stress or the imbalanced gastrointestinal system? Does stress cause a gastrointestinal system to become imbalanced, or is an imbalanced gastrointestinal system more affected by stress than a balanced one? Do you really think you've endured so much stress that your gastrointestinal system has become imbalanced and decided to seek revenge by inflicting upon you the myriad symptoms you've been experiencing? Do you think that as an additional insult, it has decided to cooperate even less when you're under the most stress? Or, was there another reason your gastrointestinal system went out of balance? Combine the imbalance with stress and your gastrointestinal system goes crazy, with your symptoms flaring. Let's say it another way: Stress only exacerbates the symptoms associated with an unhealthy gastrointestinal system. Period! Conversely, if you have a healthy, balanced gastrointestinal system, you will find yourself affected by stress in a completely different way. In fact, your gastrointestinal system may not revolt at all, or at the very least, it won't revolt as much.

The proof of this for me is that I never take level of stress into consideration when treating the patients in my office. You will never hear me say, "I'm sorry, but I think your life is too stressful and I won't be able to help you." I treat all people without regard to stress level, and everyone improves in my practice.

Furthermore, former patients who've had their beneficial bacteria population reestablished and their chemistry restored never tell me that everything is great except in times of stress. In fact, they tell me just the opposite. They say that even in stressful situations, their gastrointestinal systems don't revolt the way they used to.

Abnormal Laboratory Findings

Conventional medical doctors and researchers, when confronted with a health problem, usually try to test the affected organ or organ system to determine what physiological functions or chemistry markers are out of their "normal" ranges. If the heart is the issue, they look at cardiac output, blood pressure, cholesterol levels, and heart enzymes. If the liver is the problem, they again look at enzymes. If the brain is the area of concern, they test brain chemistry and cognitive function, and may employ computerized axial tomography (CAT scanning) or magnetic resonance imaging (MRI).

The same is true if the gastrointestinal system is the culprit. An organ system of such enormous size and importance has a lot of things that can go wrong. Luckily, doctors also have a good number of chemical markers they can check and tests they can run. A colonoscopy can detect cancer, polyps, and areas of inflammation. An endoscopy (a camera snaked down the throat into the stomach) can find ulcers and other areas of inflammation. Other tests determine if too much or too little hydrochloric acid is being produced in the stomach, how quickly the stomach empties of food, how long it takes food to transit the entire length of the system (gut motility), and how well the gallbladder and pancreas are functioning.

Much of the research that has been conducted on the gastrointestinal system has been centered on the findings that most people with IBS also suffer from impaired gut motility,

Mind-Body Connection

A very interesting concept concerns the existence of an embryological connection between the brain and the gastrointestinal system. An embryological connection is a hard wiring in the body that formed before birth. I'm sure you've heard of the mind-body connection. It's this mind-body connection that makes people think that stress is the cause of IBS.

In an embryo, groups of cells continually divide to become the very complex structures that make up a fully developed human ready for birth. At a certain point in its development, the embryo takes a C position, which resembles what we call the fetal position. Along the back side of the C is a structure called the neural tube, and what's interesting from the mind-body perspective is that two thirds of the tissue of the neural tube, which becomes more complex with each division of cells, develops into the brain and spinal cord in the fully formed human. The remaining one third develops into the nerves that connect the spinal cord to the small intestine.

There's your mind-body connection. Now you can explain to your family why they shouldn't argue during meals.

Laboratory Chemistry Makers

There are many different chemistry markers of inefficient gastrointestinal function. In addition to impaired gut motility, visceral hypersensitivity, and decreased serotonin levels, a physician can order stool testing that examines specific chemistry markers that help determine imbalances. These specific chemistry markers include normal and abnormal organisms in the gut, digestion/absorption, gut immunology, gut metabolism, enzyme levels, and fecal fats and other metabolic byproducts.

Digestion/Absorption

Pancreatic elastase and chymotrypsin are markers of digestive enzyme secretion.

Gut Immunology

Eosinophil protein X is a marker of inflammation and is elevated in food allergies, celiac sprue, and parasite infection. Calprotectin is also a marker of inflammation and is elevated in IBD, IBS, cancer, infection, food allergies, and excessive NSAID use.

Gut Metabolism

Markers such as short-chain fatty acids, n-butyrate, pH, and beta-glucuronidase suggest whether levels of beneficial bacteria are sufficient. Their metabolic activity is important for mucous production, vitamin synthesis, and detoxification of steroid hormones and bile acids.

(Continued on page 13)

a condition in which food transits the gastrointestinal system too slowly or too quickly; visceral hypersensitivity, a condition in which the nerves attached to the gut that react to stress are overly sensitive; and decreased levels of serotonin, the chemical, produced in the tissue of the gastrointestinal system, that is most responsible for preventing depression and maintaining our sense of well-being.

And again we come to the question: What came first? Did something happen to you that caused you to develop a slow or fast transit time, visceral hypersensitivity, or decreased serotonin levels, and then you developed your IBS symptoms? Or, did you lose your bacterial balance, which caused your chemistry to change, which led to your gastrointestinal system becoming unhealthy and showing abnormal test findings?

I'm sure you know by now what I believe. Proof again for me is that if slow or fast transit time, visceral hypersensitivity, and decreased serotonin levels were issues unto themselves, my protocol to reestablish proper bacterial balance and restore chemistry would never eliminate IBS symptoms. Instead, almost every one of my patients who uses my protocol sees a complete elimination of symptoms, and my guess is that if I retested these people for slow or fast transit time, visceral hypersensitivity, and decreased serotonin levels, the results would show they had returned to normal.

Genetics

Within each of us lies the potential for health or a lack of health. Which one we experience depends on the selections we make throughout life in regard to our overall environment and, more specifically, our nutritional environment. For example, some women have the gene for breast cancer but never suffer from the disease. Other people have genes for high cholesterol or heart disease but don't experience either of these chronic health conditions. The one main influence to which we all must expose our genes is the environment we create within our bodies by the foods we eat.

The new field of study called nutrigenomics examines how diet influences genetic expression and, ultimately, overall health. In other words, a bad gene will not necessarily express itself and cause a disease or health condition. It must first be exposed to variables that will cause it to express itself in the manner of a disease or health condition.

I don't know how many times patients have explained to me that their sibling, parent, or grandparent has

(Continued from page 12)

Fecal Fat Distribution

Total fecal fats is the total of triglycerides, cholesterol, phospholipids, and long-chain fatty acids. They are markers of dietary intake, digestion, and absorption.

Other Metabolic Byproducts

Percentages of acetate, propionate, and n-butyrate are markers of proper fermentation of fibers in the gastrointestinal system. Though they are useful markers to confirm the lack of balance and health that can be found in a patient's gastrointestinal tract, I never look at them. I used to test for them, but I came to realize that all patients who complain of gastrointestinal symptoms will have some of these markers out of balance.

When I used to test pre-treatment and post-treatment, I found it was apparent that the way to getting these markets back into balance is the use of the protocol presented in this book. In time, I decided the test was a waste of my patients' money.

their same symptoms, so the problem must be genetic. "Is there any hope?" they always ask. Of course, there's hope, I answer. The gastrointestinal condition may have a genetic component to it, but if we address the variables that have allowed these genes to express themselves, we will have a solution.

We're back to the old story about the loss of the bacterial balance in the gut causing, over time, a change in the chemical environment within the gut, which leads to the development of IBS symptoms. And what altered the bacterial balance and set this cascade of events into motion? Antibiotics, another environmental variable! And what do you and your sibling, parent, and maybe even grandparent all have in common? You all took antibiotics and set off the "bad" genes. And remember that antibiotics aren't the only cause, just the primary cause. Other factors that all humans share can contribute to why you and your relatives have symptoms (variables) associated with the gastrointestinal system that caused your genes to turn on you.

The next generation of holistic and alternative physicians will investigate health concerns using genetic testing, determining whether or not a person has "bad" genes and then treating that person using dietary manipulation and nutritional supplementation.

So, let's get back to the basics. Nothing fancy is going on. Don't worry about stress or genetics. You can't do anything about them anyway. Just listen to your good ol' down-home common sense, which is telling you somewhere, deep in the back of your mind, that you know something specific is causing your problem.

WHAT IBS IS

I can't tell you how many times I've heard people say they have gastrointestinal problems but they didn't know they had IBS. Many people suffer for many years, going from doctor to doctor, when suddenly one doctor finally diagnoses them with IBS. Why weren't these people diagnosed with IBS from the start? If you have a cough, you know you have a cough. If you have asthma or a headache, you know it. Why the confusion surrounding the diagnosis of IBS?

Where did the name "irritable bowel syndrome" come from? You can be sure it was coined by conventional medical people. According to the medical mindset, all symptoms and sets of symptoms must have names. How in the world can the pharmaceutical companies develop medications for things that don't have names?

It's easy to understand where the "irritable bowel" part of the name came from, but it's a little more difficult to understand why the word "syndrome" began to be used. According to the dictionaries, a syndrome is a number of symptoms occurring together and characterizing a specific disease. First of all, IBS is not a disease. It's a condition. Furthermore, IBS is not characterized by a single symptom or a specific set of symptoms. It expresses itself in a wide variety of symptoms, with different combinations of these symptoms occurring in different people. The specific symptoms a person experiences depends on that person's particular genetic strengths and weaknesses and biochemical individuality. This leads to confusion, because if you have one set of symptoms and a friend of yours has a different set of symptoms, do you both have IBS? If another friend has just one uncomfortable symptom, does that person have IBS? The answer is that all of you have IBS, but more importantly, that all of you have symptoms that you really wish would go away.

My definition of IBS is: Any uncomfortable single symptom or set of symptoms associated with the gastrointestinal tract. The possible symptoms include the following:

- ✓ Gas
- ✓ Bloating
- ✓ Indigestion
- ✓ Heartburn
- ✓ Reflux (backflow of small amounts of food from the stomach to the esophagus)
- ✓ Gastroesophageal reflux disease (GERD)
- ✓ Nausea
- ✓ Vomiting
- ✓ Diarrhea
- ✓ Constipation
- ✓ Alternating diarrhea and constipation
- ✓ Abnormal bowel frequency
- ✓ Abnormal bowel urgency
- ✓ Incomplete evacuation
- ✓ Cramping
- ✓ Sense of fullness

- ✓ Hemorrhoids

- ✓ Anal fissures (cracking of the skin of the anus)

- ✓ Fistulas

- ✓ Anal itching

- ✓ Mouth sores

- ✓ Ulcers in any part of the gastrointestinal tract

- ✓ Pain

- ✓ Gastritis (inflammation of the stomach lining)

- ✓ Esophagitis (inflammation of the esophagus)

- ✓ Gallstones or poorly functioning gallbladder

Any single symptom or combination of symptoms from this list can create discomfort. For some people, the only symptom may be diarrhea, while other people may have diarrhea, gas, bloating, and heartburn. Some people may have a combination of constipation and reflux, while still others have just a lot of embarrassing gas. Doctors only need to listen to their patients' complaints. They really don't need to give the complaints a name.

YOUR STORY

You are not alone. Most IBS sufferers travel a common path as they try to figure out—either by themselves or with the help of a conventional medical doctor—what's wrong with them. Reviewing this path will help you see that your frustration is justified. It will also help you see that your frustration has also been a good thing, since it has led you to continue looking and fighting for the solution that you know is out there.

The Path Well Traveled

It begins with a new pain, some stomach gurgling, a little heartburn, maybe gas and bloating you never had before, or a change in bowel habits. You don't really take too much notice at first. You can live with it. It's not a big deal.

Zelnorm

For the last few years, a new medication for IBS with constipation called Zelnorm has been marketed. Interestingly, it's only for women because no one has taken the time to test it on men! What? The studies found that this medication outperformed placebo in reducing discomfort associated with constipation after a trial of three months.

The FDA has approved the drug for the short-term treatment of constipation in women. How many people only have constipation for the short term? Also, aren't half of all sufferers men? What are they to do? As a side note, the researchers mentioned the medication was more effective after the first month than after three months, suggesting its benefits decrease over time.

Additionally, as of March 2007, the FDA has requested that Zelnorm be pulled from the US market citing new evidence it raised risk of heart attacks and strokes.

The bottom line is that the drug manufacturers are guessing at ways to mask the symptoms of IBS, once again not getting to the cause of the problem.

off with a prescription for Prilosec (as of 2007, available over-the-counter) or stronger prescription Nexium. Did you know that the most common side effects of Nexium are headaches, diarrhea, and abdominal pain? What are the medical experts thinking? Though the use of antacids seems reasonable and safe, these products have side effects, which I will discuss in Chapter 3.

If your complaint is diarrhea or loose bowel movements, you guzzle Imodium or Pepto-Bismol. If it's constipation, you reach for Haley's M-O, Metamucil, Citrucel, or Fibercon, and a stool softener. Fiber products are usually not high in quality, using raw materials that tend to be rough on the insides of the digestive tract, and can escort nutrition out of the body. This causes a malabsorption problem, which can have long-term consequences. If your constipation continues, you're off to your friendly doctor again, this time for Propulsid or the latest ineffective solution.

Somewhere along the way, you realize that certain foods exacerbate your problem, and you begin to avoid them or become afraid to eat. You may become afraid to leave the house, and when you do, you make sure you know the location of every bathroom between your home and your destination.

If pain is among your symptoms, you take aspirin, ibuprofen, or another non-steroidal anti-inflammatory drug (NSAID). NSAIDs are the second most common over-the-counter medication sold today. Regular use of aspirin or NSAIDs can damage the gastrointestinal system. (For a discussion of this, see "Use of Prescription and Over-the-Counter Medications" in Chapter 3.)

Since none of these over-the-counter or prescription medications or dietary changes solves your problem, you're off to your favorite well-intentioned physician once more. By now, your doctor is probably tired of seeing someone that he or she doesn't really have the tools or knowledge to help, so he or she refers you to a gastroenterologist.

The Good News/Bad News Trip to the Gastroenterologist

Gastroenterologists are specialists in the intestinal tract. They're trained to perform surgery and unique testing to rule out more serious conditions, including cancer. However, IBS usually escapes them. If you make an appointment with a gastroenterologist, you stand a good chance of walking away with a recommendation for a treatment that falls within their area of expertise. In other words, the gastroenterologist is most likely going to recommend testing or surgery.

The tests your gastroenterologist may recommend include a colonoscopy, an endoscopy, a barium enema, an MRI, and a CAT scan. By the end of your experience, you'll have been tested up this way and down that way, just to receive your first good news/bad news—all the tests came back negative, which is great because it means you're going to live, but is bad because you still have nothing to hang your hat on. And whatever's been wrong with you is still wrong.

Now you're in position for your gastroenterologist to recommend removing your gallbladder. Your gastroenterologist is a surgeon, after all, and since nothing has been found that explains your pain and other symptoms, and since an unhealthy gallbladder may cause the type of discomfort you're experiencing, he or she feels that removing the gallbladder is logical. Furthermore, as the medical profession foolishly believes, you don't really need your gallbladder. But you also better get ready for your second good news/bad news. You'll be told that your surgery went well, which I guess means you didn't die, but you'll also soon discover that you would be the rare exception if you finally found relief from your symptoms. If you experience relief, it might be temporary.

So your search continues.

Antidepressants—Even Though You're Not Depressed

More time goes by, and you try to cope as best you can after being told that you will just have to learn to live with your symptoms. But many people, especially women, find one more surprise thrown at them as they make their way along the conventional medical path. Continued visits to your favorite physician to make the same complaint over and over again result in an unspoken, industry-wide red flag that you need a prescription for an antidepressant or a referral to psychological counseling. This is a veiled medical insult. If your doctors recommend this, they are saying that they have no idea how to help you, but this can't possibly be their fault. You're a little too emotional, a little too tense, so you should just calm down, go home, and feel better about feeling so bad. Who wouldn't be tense living with IBS?

What a journey! You've gotten no results, your quality of life has continued to deteriorate, you might now be on an antidepressant that you don't need, and your money is flying out the window. You also believe that all the prescription and over-the-counter medications you've been taking are safe. After all, they've all been approved by the Food and Drug Administration (FDA). Unfortunately, all prescription and over-the-counter medications have side effects and unintended consequences.

Such a bleak picture! Could your doctor be right? IBS has no cure, and you must learn to live with your symptoms? Of course not! The answer is simple. All that doctors need to do is look back to the biochemistry, endocrinology, and physiology courses they took in medical school, plus take some nutrition courses. These courses hold the key to successfully treating IBS.

Any way you look at it, for our purposes and the purpose of this book, it's all IBS. Even if you have celiac disease, Crohn's disease, or any type of colitis, you started out with IBS.

In this chapter, we've learned that IBS isn't caused by stress, just exacerbated by it. It has genetic influences, but we can moderate those influences by addressing the variables that determine how they're expressed. We've also recognized that IBS is certainly not in your head and, even more important, that you're not alone in your struggle. We've also seen that although prestigious researchers have found abnormal laboratory findings associated with IBS, they've never been able to explain the reason for these findings or for your symptoms and discomfort.

Now that we have a clear definition of IBS, we can move on to Chapter 2 and discuss why your doctor doesn't know the information you are about to learn in the rest of this book.

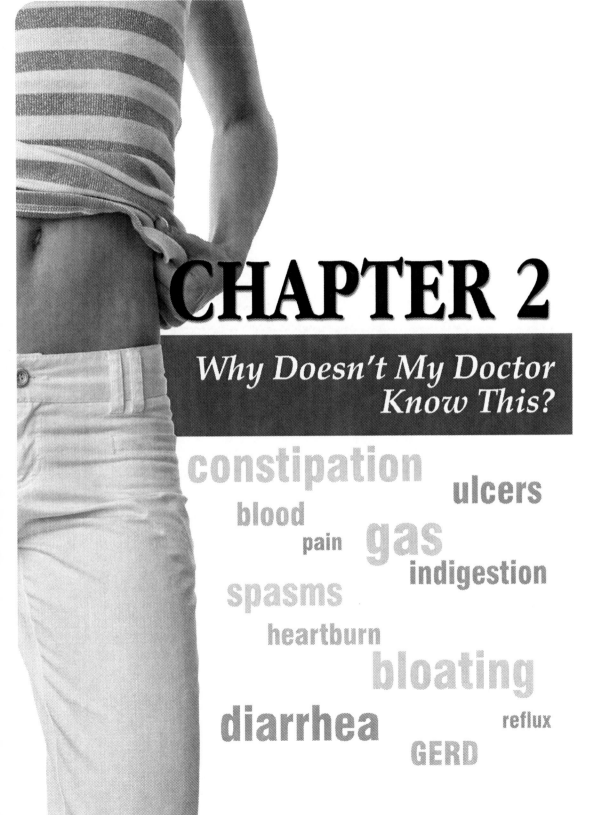

CHAPTER 2

Why Doesn't My Doctor Know This?

constipation

ulcers

blood

pain

gas

indigestion

spasms

heartburn

bloating

diarrhea

reflux

GERD

The title of this chapter is the question I'm asked most often in my office. It comes from angry, frustrated people who have just realized how sensible my explanation is about IBS—what it is, why they have it, and what they can do about it. They feel they played around with excessive tests and inappropriate treatments for too long. In this chapter, I'll answer the title question for you.

IT'S THE MEDICAL SCHOOLS' FAULT

Poor young medical students. They walk in the first day, and find that the pens, pencils, notebooks—even the clocks on the walls!—all display pharmaceutical company logos or pre-scription medication names. The indoctrination begins on day one, and it doesn't end. Never taught the critical-thought process that would help lead any human being to a rational and logical conclusion concerning why a body isn't working properly, most medical students (not all) are satisfied to learn how the body works. They then promptly forget these lessons upon graduation and reduce themselves to being pill dispensers, using as a guide what they learned from the latest pharmaceutical company representative to pay them a sales call.

The medical schools also conveniently exclude nutritional courses from their curricula, or teach very little about the subject. The names of all the B vitamins and the fact that menopausal women need extra calcium is the extent of the nutritional education at most medical schools. Some schools offer no courses, some offer one or two courses, and some progressive schools offer courses as electives. As a result, most medical students feel they have no need to know about alternative or nutritional therapies, especially when they can just dispense medications.

IT'S THE PHARMACEUTICAL COMPANIES' FAULT

Pharmaceutical companies are billion-dollar businesses. There's nothing wrong with that; this is America.

Let's see, if you and I started a pharmaceutical company, we would need three things to stay in business and remain profitable.

❖ *Perpetual research and development of new medications (products).* First and foremost, we'd need something to sell. The research and development budgets of pharmaceutical companies are gigantic. In developing our products, we'd need to keep just one concept in mind: all that our products would need to do is suppress the symptoms of health conditions, to give the appearance that they're managing the conditions, so the doctors prescribing them could look good. In a few years, we could announce breakthroughs, leading to second generations of our medications, for which we could charge more. Cures we wouldn't need.

❖ *A large sales force to teach the dispensers what to dispense.* Second, we'd need to hire a large sales force to contact all the doctors out there and teach them what they would need to know to recommend (write prescriptions for) our products. We would, of course, reward them with two-hour seminars during week-long vacations in exotic locations. The doctors who prescribed our products would further benefit because they wouldn't have to spend time critically thinking their way through a process to understand the causes of chronic health conditions.

❖ *Repeat customers.* Third, we'd need repeat customers. So, we wouldn't need to develop medications that actually cured people. If we did, we'd lose our customers.

My words are certainly harsh. And I'm probably wrong. No one who runs a pharmaceutical company thinks that way—at least, I hope not—but doesn't it seem like they do? Can you name any cures offered by conventional medicine? Antibiotics are the most obvious answer (and we know what their side effects are), possibly followed by some cancer treatments. But what else? I can't name any. More than half of the top ten chronic health conditions are diet-related. All the medications for them simply suppress the symptoms. How can you tell? If you stop taking these medications, the symptoms return and you're back to square one.

The pharmaceutical companies have too much influence on the way conventional medical doctors practice medicine, and though I may be wrong, they don't always have the best interests of the patients topmost in mind.

IT'S THE INSURANCE COMPANIES' FAULT

Insurance companies also have much too much influence on the practice of medicine. They dictate the care that their policyholders can get from their doctors. And the care they prefer is medication-related. The idea of an insurance company paying for an alternative form of medicine is completely foreign. The public is beginning to demand that this be changed, however, and thankfully, it is changing a little bit with each passing day. But for now, doctors still must stay within the guidelines of what is considered "standard medical practice" in order to get paid by the insurance companies. Only very unusual doctors operate outside the parameters.

IT'S THE DOCTORS' FAULT

From poor young medical students to poor doctors. Overworked, underpaid (in many instances), and trying to cope with insurance regulations. What doctors have the time to learn about anything new that might actually serve their patients' best interests? Indoctrinated in school, pressured by pharmaceutical reps, and restricted by insurance company guidelines. Can you blame them? I can.

Try this experiment the next time you go to your doctor. When the doctor comes in to your examining room for your four-to-six-minute consultation, reach into the pocket of his or her white coat, remove the prescription pad, and toss it into the wastebasket. Now explain your problem and see what he or she has to offer. Nothing.

And amazingly, I can't count the number of times patients have told me that their doctor or gastroenterologist said to them—with a straight face—that diet is playing no role in their IBS, Crohn's disease, or colitis symptoms. Here are specialists in the gastrointestinal system, the part of the body that processes food, who, when presented with a patient complaining of gastrointestinal symptoms, don't believe that the food the patient is eating has any relevance to the patient's symptom profile. Unbelievable!

The Hippocratic Oath requires a doctor to first do no harm. Check *Physician's Desk Reference* or read the inserts that come with your medications, and you will learn about the side effects to which you've been exposing yourself. All medications have side effects. I believe that all doctors have a moral obligation to try to help their patients from a natural perspective. The problem is that they're not taught to think that way. They're taught to suppress symptoms, not to find causes. It becomes routine for them, but at great risk to their patients.

IT'S THE CONVENTIONAL MEDICAL ESTABLISHMENT'S FAULT

"Narcissism" is defined as self-love. It's an excessive interest in one's own appearance, comfort, importance, and abilities. In Greek mythology, Narcissus was a young man who lost himself staring at his reflection in a pond. He was so in his love with his own reflection that he neither saw nor heard anything else, including the calls of a beautiful nymph named Echo. Eventually, he disturbed the water in the pond, which caused his reflection (image) to disappear. He began to grieve the loss of his reflection (image), and when Echo returned, she found nothing but a flower where Narcissus had been. Narcissus had died, lost in his love for his own reflection and in his grief over the loss of his image in the pond.

This story could be retold featuring today's conventional medical establishment, which has lost itself through its constant and narcissistic focus on its image. Conventional Medicine is so in love with itself that it sees and hears nothing else, including the calls of the beautiful nymph Alternative Medicine. Eventually, Conventional Medicine damages its image (reflection) to such an extent that it begins to grieve the loss of that image. Alternative Medicine returns, as it always does, and finds that Conventional Medicine has died, lost in its love of its own image (reflection).

Doesn't the medical community seem narcissistic? So many conventional medical doctors act like they know it all, don't accept ideas from outside their own education, and force their patients to work around their rules and schedules. Worse, if they can't seem to help a certain patient, they claim it can't be their fault. Rather, they say, it's the patient's fault!

IT'S NOT YOUR FAULT

But while your doctor may claim that it's your fault if you don't experience relief or a cure, it's not. It used to be—that is, we were all brought up to trust anything doctors told us to do, so we followed their advice blindly. But now, you're beginning to question your doctors. For one thing, you're reading this book.

So, it's not your fault anymore. In 1992, the first study found that driven by women, the number of visits to alternative health practitioners and the amount of money spent on alternative therapies began to surpass the number of visits to conventional medical doctors and the amount of money spent on conventional treatments. That was fifteen years ago and the numbers have continued to increase. This scares the heck out of the conventional medical world, and has given rise to the pseudo holistic centers that have appeared…and failed…in many local hospitals.

I know I was a little rough in this chapter on our well-intentioned conventional medical doctors. So, let's be fair. I differentiate between doctors who blindly treat chronic health conditions using the failed concept of symptom suppression and all the rest of the doctors.

Let's face it. In the United States, we have the finest acute-care doctors, emergency-room doctors, and surgeons in the world. If you break your leg, are hurt in a car accident, or need surgery, you'll get the best medical care. Medications, even with all their side effects, are necessary in many cases. I'm not against the use of medications. I'm against the *unnecessary* use of medications. There's a difference.

My problem with conventional medical doctors is restricted to the way they treat *chronic* health conditions, their lack of initiative in searching for the causes of these conditions, and their resistance to treating them using alternative medicine.

And I take it personally. Everyday I have to talk to patients whose quality of life changed dramatically because of the inabilities of conventional medicine. I see how their lives have been affected and how they've been left with no hope and nowhere to turn. Some manage to get by; others go on disability; many break into tears in my office, as they believe I may be their last hope. This isn't how medicine should be treating people. There are alternatives to conventional medical care.

Now, however, let's stop blaming the medical schools, pharmaceutical companies, and insurance companies for your continued symptoms. Let's stop being so harsh on the conventional medical doctors to whom you've turned for help. Instead, let's now turn our focus on you. In Chapter 3, I'll go into detail about the lifestyle influences that lead to IBS. Let's begin.

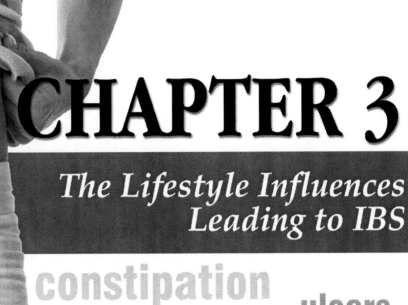

CHAPTER 3

The Lifestyle Influences Leading to IBS

constipation

ulcers

blood

pain

gas

indigestion

spasms

heartburn

bloating

diarrhea

reflux

GERD

WHY DOESN'T MY DOCTOR KNOW THIS?

Conquering Irritable Bowel Syndrome, Inflammatory Bowel Disease, Crohn's Disease, and Colitis

*T*he reason you've probably had such a frustrating experience trying to understand and overcome your symptoms is that the causes of IBS are complex. Conventional medical doctors don't do very well when it comes to dealing with multiple causes for what they perceive to be a single condition. If it's a single condition, it must have a single cause. With so many symptoms, so many combinations of symptoms, and the diverse ways patients describe their symptoms, is it any wonder conventional medical doctors can't make heads or tails out of the problem?

It's because of the medical model. Conventional doctors want to use a single molecule (medication) to suppress a single chemical process in the body and "cure" a single condition. That's why they prescribe one medicine for diarrhea, another for constipation, another for gas, another for nausea, and yet another to prevent heartburn. The complex reasons that cause all of these problems in the same person escape most conventional medical doctors, and the inability of most doctors to critically think through all of the clues that point to the causes is conventional medicine's biggest failing.

In this chapter, we'll discuss the many potential lifestyle influences that lead to IBS. Most people have contact with each of these influences at some time. The use of antibiotics is the primary influence, the one that sets into motion the cascade of events that ultimately leads to the loss of balance in your gastrointestinal system. It's not the only reason, however. We'll also cover the secondary influences leading to IBS that might have contributed to the overall loss of balance in your system.

THE PRIMARY LIFESTYLE INFLUENCE LEADING TO IBS

My premise is that the lifestyle factors that influence IBS and the treatment of IBS are both complex but, at the same time, very simple. I believe both revolve around bacteria and chemistry.

Case History: Carrie

Carrie, a 43-year-old female complaining of diarrhea and embarrassing gas and bloating, came to my office to discuss whether or not my IBS protocol might help her. I explained to her my focus on antibiotics affecting bacterial levels and the subsequent changes to the chemistry of the gastrointestinal system. She wanted to participate in parts of my protocol, but as a cost saving measure, she opted to skip taking the probiotics I recommended because she insisted she had used only a couple of courses of antibiotics in her lifetime, so that couldn't be her problem.

Because of her stance, I ordered a stool test to be taken to identify the levels of beneficial bacteria and any abnormal bacteria or yeast (see Laboratory Tests in the Resource List at the back of this book). What was revealed changed her mind and reinforced something I have told my patients for years.

The lab reported very low amounts of *Lactobacillus acidophilus* and *Bifidus*. In fact, her levels were so low, the lab reported them as NG (no growth). We added the probiotics to her treatment plan, and within days she experienced changes and within a few weeks her bowel movements were normal and the gas and bloating nonexistent.

I have said for years that it doesn't matter if people have had two or two hundred courses of antibiotics in their lifetime or whether they haven't taken them for many years. Any time you take them, they will alter or damage the optimal levels of beneficial bacteria.

Once a body's beneficial bacteria levels are altered, its chemistry will begin to change and, over time, it will develop symptoms. The primary reason—though not the only reason—bacteria levels become altered is the use of antibiotics. Designed to kill the bacterial infections that cause illnesses such as sore throat, ear infection, bronchitis, and urinary tract infection, antibiotics unfortunately also destroy a portion of the good bacteria living in the gastrointestinal system, causing the ratio of good bacteria to bad bacteria to change for the worse. It doesn't matter how many courses of antibiotics you've taken over your lifetime or when you took them. Each time you took an antibiotic, you altered the balance of good to bad bacteria that's so important for human health and proper gastrointestinal function.

Are you aware that the insert that comes along with prescription antibiotics, describing the medication and its action, warns that its use "alters the normal flora of the colon"? You never read the insert that closely, did you? If you're like me, your answer is no. The insert goes on to say that an abnormal growth of bad bacteria may then follow the loss of the good bacteria. This information is also listed for antibiotics in *Physician's Desk Reference*, the medical profession's compilation of data on prescription medications.

When your bacteria levels are imbalanced, the potential for the bad bacteria already present in your system to overgrow their normal levels or for you to pick up additional bad bacteria from contaminated food or water, your pets, another human, or an unsanitary environment is greatly enhanced. In a healthy gastrointestinal system with proper beneficial bacteria levels, potentially problematic organisms may never gain a foothold. In other words, they could be transient, causing a temporary problem or no problem at all.

Antibiotic use begins a slow, slippery slide into losing the health of your gastrointestinal tract, and the situation can be further complicated if you come into contact with other organisms that would love to live inside you. People with IBS need to reestablish their beneficial bacteria levels. If they've picked up hitchhikers—and I find that about 30 percent of my patients generally have—they need to take measures to eliminate them. The good news is that it's easy to reestablish the proper bacterial balance in people with IBS, and I'll describe how to do this in Chapter 4.

SECONDARY LIFESTYLE INFLUENCES LEADING TO IBS

The use of antibiotics is certainly enough to unbalance your gastrointestinal system and create the environment for IBS. Couple their use with secondary lifestyle influences, and you stand an even greater chance of losing health in your gastrointestinal tract and eventually suffering from symptoms.

Lack of Digestive Enzymes

If your symptoms include gas, bloating, indigestion, heartburn, reflux, GERD, pain, or cramps, your problem usually is the consumption of foods you don't tolerate well (see Chapter 5) coupled with a lack of digestive enzymes, such as hydrochloric acid (stomach acid) or pancreatic enzymes, especially the older we get.

Digestion actually begins in the mouth, where food is chewed, resulting in more surface area for the enzymes to work on. Salivary amylase, an enzyme secreted with the saliva, helps to break apart the food and begins the digestion of starches. In the stomach, hydrochloric acid is released and begins the digestion of proteins. After the food moves from the stomach to the intestines, the pancreas kicks in with a full complement of enzymes, including protease, for protein digestion; more amylase, for starch and carbohydrate digestion; and lipase, for fat digestion. The gallbladder squeezes out bile, which boosts the effect of the lipase and assists with the fat digestion. The small intestine also secretes a number of enzymes that assist in the digestive process.

The digestive enzyme most people seem to know is hydrochloric acid. People who have heartburn, reflux, or GERD usually think they have too much stomach acid. That's why they take Tums, Rolaids, Pepcid AC, Tagamet, Prilosec, or Nexium. But if you ask a gastroenterologist, you'll learn that in reality, very few people produce too much stomach acid. In fact, many people actually produce too little. "Sure, Doc, that's great," you might say, "but that can't be me because I feel the acid. It burns and hurts, and it comes up into my throat. I must be the exception." The odds are you're not.

If you ask a physician or nurse to name the symptoms of producing too much stomach acid, they will quickly list the symptoms I mentioned above. But if you ask that same physician or nurse to name the symptoms of producing too little stomach acid, you'll probably get silence. It's because most conventional medical doctors and nurses don't realize that the symptoms of producing too little stomach acid are exactly the same as those of producing too much. How do you know which category you fall into? Have you diagnosed yourself? Do the three or four commercials you see every night while watching television have you convinced that you need an antacid for your symptoms? "Yeah, but Doc, when I take an antacid, I feel better," you might say.

Well, some people do. Some people find permanent relief through taking antacids, and some people get temporarily relief, until the antacid stops working. But one thing all these people have in common is that antacids don't cure their problems. Many people with IBS have taken antacids for years or even decades. They have bottles in their kitchens, bathrooms, offices, and automobiles. Antacids merely suppress symptoms. If these people stop taking their antacids, they find they still have their same problems. But wait. There's worse news.

Antacids buffer away the acid the stomach has produced, thereby decreasing the pH of the stomach content, and since most people don't produce enough acid anyway, this creates an even greater inability to break down proteins. As if that weren't bad enough, a lowered level of hydrochloric acid in the stomach inhibits minerals such as calcium, magnesium, and potassium from being properly prepared for later absorption in the small intestine. And if that's still not bad enough, acid is a potent weapon in the fight against food-borne bacteria. Buffer it away, and you greatly increase your chances of developing food poisoning or having abnormal bacteria take hold in your gastrointestinal tract. On top of it all, the antacid manufacturers have the nerve to supplement their products with the poorest quality calcium known to man and to then act as if they're doing you a favor!

The bottom line is that too many people take antacids because they think that their bodies are producing too much acid (which they aren't) and that antacids will solve the problem (which they won't). In reality, antacids inhibit the process of digestion and prevent the proper absorption of minerals in the small intestine. If you take antacids, you therefore also don't get all the available nutrition from your food.

Here's why most people think they're producing too much stomach acid. A sphincter muscle at the bottom of the esophagus is supposed to close and prevent the acid that's in the stomach from splashing into the esophagus. If your sphincter muscle isn't working properly, it doesn't matter if you're producing too little or too much stomach acid. Whatever acid is in your stomach can splash past the sphincter muscle onto the base of your unprotected esophagus. The stomach is protected from the acid by a coating of mucus, but the esophagus is not.

One of the main reasons that any muscle—and specifically, the sphincter muscle—doesn't work properly is calcium deficiency. Didn't I just mention taking antacids prevents the proper absorption of minerals like calcium in the small intestine? Could there be a connection?

Use of Prescription and Over-the-Counter Medications

We live in a society that thinks it can solve its problems with pills. We are constantly exposed to advertisements in newspapers and magazines, on television and radio, and even on our computers for over-the-counter medications. Advertising works. Therefore, we all self-medicate.

What could possibly be wrong with an aspirin? If we have a headache, we reach for one. If it's a bad headache, or if we have aches and pains along with the headache, we might choose Tylenol, Advil, Motrin, or something similar. If we have a cough, we take cough syrup. If we have sinus congestion, with drainage down the back of the throat or out the nose, we take a decongestant and antihistamine. They stop you right up.

How about something to help you sleep or wake up? For diarrhea? For constipation?

Did you ever stop and think that there might be a reason you have a headache, a cough, sinus drainage? Is your body trying to accomplish something? Might these symptoms be normal reactions? Coughing helps clear the lungs. Sinus drainage gets rid of unwanted mucus harboring germs. Diarrhea clears anything unwanted from the bowels. Should we really interfere with what the body is trying to do?

Top-Selling Prescription Medications in June 2004

Lipitor (cholesterol)
Zocor (cholesterol)
Plavix (blood thinner)
Norvasc (blood pressure)
Seretide (asthma)
Ogastro (ulcers)
Effexor (antidepressant)
Zyprexa (antipsychotic)
Zoloft (antidepressant)

Additional Top Sellers
Premarin (estrogen)
Synthroid (thyroid)
Atenolol (blood pressure)
Furosemide (diuretic)
Prilosec (antacid)
Albuterol (asthma)
Xanax (anxiety)
Propoxyphene (pain)
Glucophage (diabetes)
Cephalexin (antibiotic)
Amoxicillin (antibiotic)
Claritin (allergies)
Trimax (antibiotic)
Hydrochlorothiazide (diuretic)
Zithromax (antibiotic)
Prozac (antidepressant)
Ibupropen (pain)
Paxil (antidepressant)
NSAIDs
Source: IMS Health

Do you have a headache because of a lack of Tylenol in your bloodstream? Of course not, but believe it or not, this is what some people think. Pain relievers don't cure the cause of pain. They only mask the pain, actually blocking the receptors in the body that sense pain. Some great "cure" that is.

The same way that prescription medications have side effects (with the number-one side effect being gastrointestinal problems), over-the-counter medications also have consequences. According to a report published in 1999 in the *New England Journal of Medicine*, a study conducted at Boston University School of Medicine showed "significant and potentially fatal side-effects of non-steroidal anti-inflammatory drugs (NSAIDs) such as aspirin, Advil, Motrin, Aleve, Naprosyn, Naprox, Voltaren and Indocin." The lead researcher called this a "silent epidemic," because warning signs don't precede gastrointestinal complications. What have I been saying? You may or may not have any symptoms that you can link to the use of NSAIDs. You may not even be aware of the process leading to the symptoms.

The complications to which the lead researcher referred were gastric damage, ulcers, and bleeding. These complications have also been linked to arthritis, which means that NSAIDs cause a change in chemistry that results in inflammation. The lead researcher added that these complications could be potentially fatal. Sounds extreme, doesn't it? Not when you realize that between 7,600 and 16,500 deaths occur every year from ulcer-related complications, and over 100,000 people are hospitalized each year from complications resulting from NSAIDs use. For our purposes, however, the primary thing to realize is that the use of over-the-counter medications in general and NSAIDs in particular contributes to the problem we're trying to solve.

Presence of Abnormal Bacteria, Yeast, or Parasites

The presence of abnormal bacteria, yeast, or parasites in your system will complicate your recovery from IBS because these organisms often produce their own symptoms. The most common symptoms they cause are diarrhea and gas, but because their presence means that your gastrointestinal tract isn't healthy or functioning properly, other symptoms might be related to them. The organisms need to be eliminated, and I'll describe how to do that in the section about Laboratory Tests in the Resource List at the back of this book. That section also discusses the sensitivity report usually provided by the lab that tells the practitioner what prescription medications or natural antimicrobial products to use to eliminate them.

If your doctor has already had you submit a stool sample for testing but the lab didn't find anything and you were told you have no problems, find out exactly for what your sample was tested. Conventional medical doctors typically test for the presence of blood, parasites, and parasite eggs. This is entirely useless for our purposes because rarely do we see parasites in humans in Western society. In addition, it means you weren't tested for your level of good bacteria, the more commonly found abnormal bacteria, yeast, or parasites. The good bacteria in which you would be interested are *Lactobacillus acidophilus* and *Bifidobacterium*. Abnormal bacteria or yeast consist of any that are present at levels lab criteria consider to be greater than those found in a normal gastrointestinal tract, and all parasites need to be eliminated.

The lab to which your doctor sent your sample is also very important. Local labs may be unqualified to find the organisms that could be contributing to your problem. Different labs use different techniques and have different quality-control standards. You need to use a lab that specializes in stool testing. (For laboratory recommendations, see the Laboratory Test section in the Resource List at the back of this book.)

Poor Food Choices

How many people have a perfect diet? No one does. Do you pay attention at all to what you eat? How much fast food is in your diet? How much fried food? How much milk, cheese, and ice cream? How much of your foods are processed, already prepared, and packaged? No matter what you eat, how much do you eat? Do you overeat, or do you hardly eat at all? Either way, your choices have consequences.

If you eat a lot of fast foods, highly processed foods, or foods made of white flour and sugar, you're not only starving your body in general, but you're also not providing the tissue inside your gastrointestinal system with the nutrients it needs to be healthy. Without healthy tissue, your intestines can't absorb whatever nutrients you do eat. Remember, the cause of IBS and its solution are both very much about chemistry.

The cause of IBS has been a hotly debated topic. Conventional medicine has researched the condition for years, but has never come up with any cause that people with IBS could count on. Common sense may be our best researcher when it comes to this condition. It makes sense that if humans need a population of beneficial bacteria living in their gastrointestinal systems and antibiotics destroy bacteria, then the taking of antibiotics might play a role in IBS. Conventional medicine knows this, hence the warning on the inserts accompanying all antibiotic prescriptions.

It makes sense that if you've picked up an abnormal or potentially problematic bacterium, parasite, or other organism from the environment that shouldn't be living inside the human gastrointestinal system, you need to take measures to eliminate it. It makes sense that if you're not producing enough digestive enzymes or are impairing their efficiency in any way, you may be contributing to the ability of these organisms to live inside you or properly perform their functions.

It also makes sense that if you have a history of taking prescription medications, over-the-counter medications, and especially NSAIDs, you may be experiencing side effects from them that could be contributing to your symptoms.

In this chapter, we've outlined the potential lifestyle influences leading to IBS. In Chapter 4, we'll discuss the nutrients and other substances that you can use to help reestablish a proper bacterial balance in your gut and restore normal chemistry to its tissue.

CHAPTER 4

The Supplements

constipation

ulcers

blood

pain

gas

indigestion

spasms

heartburn

bloating

diarrhea

reflux

GERD

$\mathcal{U}$nderstanding what IBS is and isn't, why your conventional medical doctor has been unable to help you, and what causes IBS is important, but not nearly as important as learning what to do about the condition. The information in this chapter may sound familiar, but please read it anyway. You might learn something new. I have many different people come into my office each day, and some of them have been searching for the information in this chapter for a very long time.

The search for a solution to their IBS symptoms begins for most people at a conventional medical doctor's office. At some point, whether after a short time or many years, the treatment becomes frustrating. The frustration typically leads people to a local bookstore, where they buy anything they can find on gastrointestinal problems in general and IBS in particular. The suggestions in these books include diets, recipes, stress reduction, exercise, massage, vitamins, herbs, homeopathy, visualization, biofeedback, reflexology, yoga, meditation, hypnotherapy, and magnets, which bring varying degrees of success.

Further exploration leads many people with IBS to a local health food store. There they receive advice from well-intentioned seven-dollar-an-hour employees who work in the store because they're "into health" and have done more reading than the average customer. Following their advice usually leads to a cupboard full of various vitamins, minerals, and herbs, along with a lighter pocketbook. Some people may find partial success, but no one ever finds a cure. Taking supplements by themselves, without a plan, is just like taking medications. Supplements aren't as toxic as medications, and they usually don't have the side effects, but taking them in isolation again just suppresses symptoms, it doesn't cure anything.

Interestingly enough, you may have already tried some of the supplements I suggest in this chapter. However, you haven't tried all of my suggestions, all at the same time, and in the order I recommend. It is the completeness of this plan that supplies the final missing pieces to the puzzle of restoration of your gastrointestinal health.

Case History: Carol

Carol was a 51-year-old female complaining of constipation, gas, and heartburn. She set an appointment to discuss her symptoms and my protocol, but was reluctant to go ahead with my protocol because she told me she thought she had already tried all the suggestions I made for her. I finally convinced her there were distinct differences between what I suggested and what she had already tried.

She was "sort of" correct in thinking some of my advice had already failed her. She had gone to a health food store and purchased some probiotics. Her symptoms never changed while she took them, so she stopped. She went back to the health food store and bought some digestive enzymes. She did notice some change in the gas and bloating she experienced, but not in the constipation or heartburn. For a short period of time, she gave up almost all dairy products. Again, she saw no positive changes.

(Continued on page 43)

By the time most people reach my office, they're worn out and frustrated, they've already spent a boatload of money, and they're wary of the next step. They're often skeptical of what I may propose to them, but they've come to me because they feel they have no other options. Frustration leads to desperation. Luckily, they've come to the right place.

Remember that you don't have a disease. You have a condition as a result of certain lifestyle influences that have caused a set of symptoms that are nothing more than your body talking to you. Your body is trying to tell you something.

In this chapter, we'll learn how to answer your body. The response begins with a number of essential supplements for an average of three months and may include some special-circumstance supplements as well. All of the supplements mentioned can be found through online sources or health food stores. Please refer to the Essential Supplements section of the Resource List at the back of this book.

ESSENTIAL SUPPLEMENTS TO REESTABLISH BACTERIAL BALANCE

Taking therapeutic dosages of beneficial bacteria is essential to begin the restoration of health in your gastrointestinal system. These beneficial bacteria must include the two major types of bacteria called *Lactobacillus* and *Bifidobacterium* (*Bifidus*). The specific *Lactobacillus* species that have proven to be the most beneficial are *L. acidophilus, L. salivarius, L. paracasei,* and *L. plantarum.* The specific *Bifidus* species that has proven to be the most beneficial is *lactis.*

Beneficial bacteria supplements, also known as probiotics, help reestablish your own genetically determined "wild type" organisms by providing the chemistry (fermentation byproducts) that will promote their growth. You originally obtained your "wild type" strains from the birth canal, your parents' (especially mother's) skin, and food.

Take the recommended beneficial bacteria supplements for three months. They need to be taken by everyone with IBS, no matter the specific symptoms.

Lactobacillus

Try to find a dairy-free supplement that includes *L. acidophilus, L. salivarius, L. paracasei,* and *L. plantarum,* as well as *Streptococcus thermophilus.* Note the specific strains the product uses because all probiotics are not created equal.

When shopping for *Lactobacillus,* make sure that the product you select is guaranteed by the manufacturer to provide no fewer than 15 billion combined live organisms per serving **through the expiration date.** Note that *Lactobacillus* needs to be refrigerated; do not purchase a product that claims not to need refrigeration.

What It Does

The *Lactobacillus* blend of probiotics primarily repopulates the small intestine. The specifically chosen organisms support a broad range of digestive and immune-system functions. We have already discussed the benefits of having a proper bacterial balance in

(Continued from page 42)

Whenever patients say they have tried most of my advice without success, I know full well they have not. The differences are many in what they have done and what I suggest. First and most important, there are many parts of my advice that must be done all at the same time. Trying some probiotics for a while, giving up, and then eliminating dairy for a while is not what I suggest. All of the supplements must be used at the same time and the dietary eliminations must be followed with them. The additional dietary eliminations, if necessary, must be done in the order outlined in the protocol.

I was finally able to convince Carol of the differences between what she had tried and what I was suggesting, and to her pleasant surprise, within a couple months she was symptom-free.

the gastrointestinal tract. Studies have shown that a lack of beneficial bacteria in the system can lead to an environment that contributes to IBS symptoms.

Using Yogurt to Reestablish Bacterial Balance

How many people do you know who eat a container of yogurt every day while taking a course of antibiotics? Some people eat yogurt every day even when not taking antibiotics. Why? The power of advertising.

Yogurt has become the method of choice in the United States for the mis-informed to attempt to reestablish and maintain bacterial balance in the gastrointestinal system. You cannot reestablish bacterial balance through the ingestion of yogurt, no matter how much acidophilus it contains. Yogurt can never come close to supplying the amount of acidophilus needed to accomplish this, especially for those suffering from IBS, Crohn's disease or any type of colitis. The reason is simple. Yogurt, by definition, contains very little acidophilus, just enough to ferment the milk into yogurt. If you analyze the name *Lactobacillus acidophilus*, you'll see that it refers to a type of organism called a bacillus, which is acid-loving (acidophilus). As *lactobacillus acidophilus* turns milk into yogurt, it creates an alkaline environment, in which it can't live. Therefore, the more the acidophilus ferment milk into yogurt, the more they cause their population to be killed off. Also note that lactobacillus acidophilus is not the only probiotic I recommend in my treatment plan.

What to Use

Lactobacillus is usually found in capsule form. Take 15 billion organisms twice a day on an empty stomach for three months. These organisms will survive contact with stomach acid if taken on an empty stomach.

Bifidobacterium

Try to find a dairy-free supplement that includes *B. lactis* and *S. thermophilus*. Note the specific strains the product uses because, as mentioned for *Lactobacillus*, all probiotics are not created equal.

When shopping for *Bifidobacterium*, make sure that the product you select is guaranteed by the manufacturer to provide no fewer than 15 billion combined live organisms per serving through the expiration date. Note that *Bifidobacterium* needs to be refrigerated; do not purchase a product that claims not to need refrigeration.

What It Does

The *Bifidobacterium* blend of probiotics promotes a healthy microbial balance primarily in the large intestine. Studies of *B. lactis* have shown that these organisms relieve minor intestinal irritation, support normal intestinal motility, and assist intestinal immune-cell function.

What to Use

Bifidobacterium is usually found in capsule form. Take 15 billion organisms twice a day, on an empty stomach for three months. These organisms will survive contact with stomach acid if taken on an empty stomach.

ESSENTIAL SUPPLEMENTS TO FEED THE TISSUE AND RESTORE CHEMISTRY

As explained in Chapter 3, once a body's bacteria levels change, the chemistry of the tissue in its gastrointestinal system also changes over time. This means that at a cellular level, the tissue probably becomes inflamed (even though no diagnosis of an inflammatory condition is made), which causes it to become inefficient at the normal task of deciding what to absorb and what to eliminate. In other words, the gastrointestinal system becomes just plain unhealthy.

Thanks to our knowledge of biochemistry and the physiology of the gastrointestinal system, we know which nutrients will feed and heal this tissue, helping it return to normal. While you usually obtain these nutrients from the food you eat as it passes through your gastrointestinal tract, you need to also take them in supplemental form, in large therapeutic dosages for three months. A unique thing about the tissue in the gastrointestinal tract is that the outside layer, the one closest to the food passing through,

You Can Be Too Clean

Since babies get their initial beneficial bacteria in part from their parents' skin, our society's fascination with antibacterial soaps can have a profound unintended consequence. How many people have antibacterial soap by their kitchen sink, every bathroom sink, and even in their car? It may seem like splitting hairs, but these soaps are unnecessary. Being too clean can be bad for both adults and children.

Bacteria are everywhere. Because of this, you need to keep some on your skin because this keeps your immune system exposed to them and therefore at its highest level of preparedness. Without bacteria present on your skin, your immune system becomes lazy and weak. If new parents don't have bacteria present on their skin, they can't provide their babies with the necessary beneficial organisms.

sloughs off every three to seven days. As you feed your system therapeutic amounts of these healing nutrients, each new layer becomes a little healthier, allowing it to absorb a greater percentage of the nutrients from food, and creating an even healthier following layer. Eventually, you will have a brand-new gastrointestinal system, one that can make better decisions about what to absorb and what to eliminate. All in all, you'll be just plain healthier.

The supplements that supply the nutrients that feed the tissue and restore proper chemistry are rice protein powder, glutamine and other amino acids, inulin, and fructo-oligosaccharides (FOS). They are best taken mixed together in the form of a drink.

Genetically Predetermined Probiotics

I am often asked where we get our population of beneficial bacteria. We are not born with it. Rather, we ingest it from our environment and, mostly, from our parents.

When a baby is born, the first contact he or she has with beneficial bacteria is in the birth canal. The same bacteria that inhabits our gastrointestinal system is on our skin, and each time the baby feeds, the bacteria from Mom's skin begins to populate his or her little gastrointestinal system. Dad also gets into the act through contact with the child, possibly by holding the baby up on his bare shoulder, where the baby licks or sucks his skin, or by putting his finger in the baby's mouth for a moment.

Another source of bacteria is raw food. Though washed, raw food still has some "good" bacteria on it.

Can you see how antibacterial soaps or being too clean can be bad for a child?

Rice Protein Powder

Rice protein powder, like whey protein powder and soy protein powder, offers a quick and convenient way to boost your daily protein intake. Often used as the base for smoothies, it can also be added to other recipes to boost the protein content. For our purposes, rice protein powder is best because whey is a dairy product (we're avoiding those) and soy powder is hard to digest and is a known allergen. Therefore, rice protein powder is better for people with IBS.

What It Does

Rice protein powder contains phytochemicals, peptides, and a complete amino acid profile, all of which have beneficial effects on the tissue lining the gastrointestinal system.

What to Use

Take 30 grams of rice protein powder mixed into water twice a day. To prepare the drink, follow the manufacturer's directions for three months.

Glutamine

Amino acids are the building blocks of protein, and glutamine is one of the more common amino acids found in the protein we eat. Used by the body for more than five hundred chemical reactions, it's also the preferred fuel for the rapidly dividing cells of the gastrointestinal lining.

What It Does

The primary purpose of glutamine in our protocol is to feed the cells that line the gastrointestinal tract. Glutamine is the main amino acid that will help the tissue that sloughs off to be replaced by healthier tissue. In addition to serving as food for the cells, glutamine also supports a healthy mucosal barrier and promotes the production of glutathione, another amino acid that supports healing and protects against oxidation.

Animal studies have shown glutamine to be important in gut immune function. Glutamine deficiency has been associated with atrophy and degenerative changes in the small intestine. Ingesting therapeutic amounts of this amino acid for a short period of time simply improves the health of the tissue of the gastrointestinal system.

What to Use

Take 500 milligrams of glutamine twice a day. For best results, add it to the rice protein drink and take for three months.

Other Amino Acids

So much of nature works in a synergistic manner. Adding additional amino acids to your rice protein drink will enhance the action of all of the amino acids it includes and will provide your gastrointestinal tissue with a more complete protein profile. The additional amino acids I recommend are N-acetylcysteine, L-glutathione, L-cysteine, L-lysine, and L-threonine.

What They Do

N-acetylcysteine, L-glutathione, and L-cysteine help to detoxify the tissue of the gastrointestinal tract. They also act as antioxidants and improve the integrity of the gut lining. L-lysine and L-threonine help to make the protein profile of the rice protein drink more complete.

What to Use

Take 5 milligrams each of N-acetylcysteine, L-glutathione, and L-cysteine and 35 milligrams each of L-lysine and L-threonine twice a day. For best results, add them to the rice protein drink and take for three months.

Inulin

Inulin is a polysaccharide (chain of sugars) that is derived from the chicory plant. It's not absorbed by the human gastrointestinal tract, but simply passes right through it.

What It Does

Inulin increases fecal bulk, helps improve the population of acidophilus and *Bifidobacterium* and improves other important chemical markers found in the gastrointestinal tract. In addition, it improves mineral absorption, assists B-vitamin synthesis by the beneficial bacteria, lowers total cholesterol and triglyceride levels, stabilizes insulin and glucose levels, and enhances immune function.

What to Use

Take 1,400 milligrams of inulin twice a day for three months. For best results, add it to the rice protein drink.

Fructo-oligosaccharides

Fructo-oligosaccharides (FOS) is a polysaccharide or short chain of sugar molecules ("oligo" means "few," and "saccharide" means "sugar"). It's a nondigestible dietary sugar that feeds the beneficial bacterial population. Its molecules are not absorbed by the human gastrointestinal tissue, but simply pass right through the body.

What It Does

FOS provides a favorite food of the beneficial bacteria that populate the human gastrointestinal system, thereby helping to increase their numbers. The beneficial bacteria also ferment FOS, which helps to improve the chemistry and the health of the entire system.

What to Use

Take 2,000 milligrams of FOS twice a day. For best results, add it to the rice protein drink and take for three months.

ESSENTIAL SUPPLEMENTS TO IMPROVE DIGESTION AND RESTORE pH

In time, on this program, you'll be able to throw away your Tums, Rolaids, Pepcid AC, Imodium, Pepto-Bismol, Nexium, and Prilosec. Impaired digestion causes many of the symptoms associated with irritable bowel syndrome. Without sufficient secretion of digestive enzymes, IBS symptoms occur. Therefore, supplementation with digestive enzymes, as well as nutrients that assist the digestive process, is an important part of our program.

The most important digestive-enzyme supplements to take for our purposes are hydrochloric acid and the pancreatic enzymes (protease, amylase, and lipase). Gas and bloating are often the result of the body's inability to break down food within a certain amount of time. Hydrochloric acid is the first major enzyme with which food comes into contact in the body (after salivary amylase, a small amount of which is secreted with the saliva in the mouth). The pancreatic enzymes follow, secreted into the food as it's released from the stomach into the upper part of the small intestine. We will add supplements of all these enzymes to each meal to make sure you have full-strength digestive ability.

Note that if you have a history of gastritis or ulcers, these products may make you uncomfortable. However, if you were diagnosed a year or more ago and addressed the problem with a doctor, I highly recommend that go ahead and use the supplements. You can follow the program without them, but your results will be better with them. If you experience discomfort, you can always stop taking them. If you progress in the program without them and the irritated areas of your gastrointestinal tract begin to heal, you'll eventually be able to add these supplements back in again.

If you've had your gallbladder removed, you will benefit from taking a combination of choline, inositol, taurine, and L-methionine. Remember that well-intentioned conventional medical doctor who explained that removing your gallbladder might relieve your symptoms? That doctor couldn't have been more wrong, huh? Now your body has problems digesting fats, which may actually be causing you to have more pain, gas, bloating and diarrhea than you had before your surgery! Don't eliminate or reduce the fats you eat as an answer to your problem. Fats are necessary for human health, and you'll suffer other consequences if you skip eating them. Instead, take the supplements I recommend to improve fat digestion—not just for the duration of this program, but forever—and you should no longer have a problem digesting the fats in your diet.

In addition to the above supplements, I also recommend taking chamomile, peppermint, and lavender, all of which are known for their soothing effects on the gastrointestinal system.

Betaine Hydrochloride

Betaine hydrochloride is the supplemental form of hydrochloric acid. Betaine is a vitamin like substance found in beets that increases the concentration of acids in the stomach. For our purposes, take the betaine hydrochloride either as part of a combination product also containing pepsin and gentian root, or take it as separate product along with pepsin and gentian root.

What It Does

The combination of betaine hydrochloride, pepsin, and gentian root assists primarily with the breakdown of proteins. In addition, the combination improves the pH in the gastrointestinal tract.

Betaine hydrochloride, which is similar to the hydrochloric acid produced in the stomach, will boost the amount of hydrochloride acid you have available for the digestion of the protein you consume. Pepsin is a proteolytic enzyme, which is a type of enzyme that breaks down proteins, and gentian root is an herbal bitter traditionally used to support healthy digestion.

What to Use

Take 1,300 milligrams of betaine hydrochloride, 90 milligrams of pepsin, and 40 milligrams of gentian root immediately after every meal or within 30 minutes of finishing the meal. Take them either in the form of a combination product or as separate products used together.

Caution

If you experience any discomfort (pain or nausea) after taking these supplements, discontinue their use. Either you don't need to boost your hydrochloric-acid content or you have an area of inflammation somewhere in your esophagus, stomach, or upper gastrointestinal tract that is being irritated. Wait two to three weeks and then try taking the supplements again. You may find the healing process that has taken place will allow you to take them without discomfort. If not, stop taking them for a month and reintroduce them again.

Also, don't make a decision not to use them because you believe you don't have a problem digesting proteins. Remember, they have the additional benefit of correcting the pH of the material moving through your system.

Pancreatic Enzymes

The pancreatic enzymes protease, amylase, and lipase taken together form a comprehensive enzyme complex just like that secreted from the pancreas. The combination helps promote healthy digestive function and also improves the pH in the gastrointestinal tract.

What They Do

Protease is the name for a group of enzymes that include chymotrypsin, trypsin, papain, pepsin and chymosin that function together to break down protein and fight inflammation. Amylase, also known as carbohydrase or glycogenase, breaks down carbohydrates, and lipase breaks down fat.

What to Use

Take 156,000 United States Pharmacopoeia (USP) units each of protease and amylase, and 24,960 USP units of lipase before (or up to thirty minutes after starting) every meal. Take them either in the form of a combination product or as separate products used together.

Caution

If you experience any discomfort (pain or nausea) after taking these supplements, discontinue their use. Either you don't need to boost your pancreatic-enzyme content or you have an area of inflammation somewhere in your esophagus, stomach, or upper gastrointestinal tract that is being irritated. Wait two to three weeks and then try taking the supplements again. You may find the healing process that has taken place will allow you to take them without discomfort. If not, stop taking them for a month and reintroduce them again.

Lipotropic Nutrients

Lipotropic nutrients are fat-digesting nutrients and highly recommended for people who have had their gallbladders removed or who have trouble digesting fats. Look for a combination product that contains choline (in the form of choline bitartrate), inositol, taurine, and L-methionine. Ideally, the product should also contain a variety of additional synergistic vitamins, minerals, and herbs, such as vitamins C, B6, and B12, folic acid, magnesium, and artichoke leaf.

What They Do

Choline is a vitamin that regulates the gallbladder and minimizes excess fat in the liver by aiding fat metabolism. Inositol, also a vitamin, functions in fat metabolism and helps to remove fats from the liver. Taurine, an amino acid, is a key component of bile, which is secreted by the liver and stored in the gallbladder, and is needed for fat digestion and absorption of the fat-soluble vitamins. The essential amino acid L-methionine assists in fat breakdown and helps to prevent fat buildup in the liver.

What to Use

Take 150 milligrams of choline bitartrate, 75 milligrams of inositol, and 50 milligrams each of taurine and L-methionine before (or up to thirty minutes after starting) every meal. Take them either in the form of a combination product or as separate products used together.

Chamomile, Peppermint, and Lavender

Specific oils from herbs are an especially effective product and work extremely well for people with malabsorption problems. The herbs are cold pressed with a heavy hydraulic press to not degrade their effectiveness.

I recommend using chamomile, peppermint, and lavender, since all three are noted for their comforting relief of gastrointestinal disturbances. This blend of oils helps relax intestinal smooth muscle (antispasmodic) and relieves symptoms of indigestion and flatulence.

What They Do

Chamomile, peppermint, and lavender as a group help to relax the smooth muscle tissue in the gastrointestinal tract to provide relief of occasional intestinal discomfort. They also support healthy colonic motility and relieve symptoms of occasional indigestion. Peppermint is an antispasmodic and reduces the production of gas. Lavender and chamomile promote relaxation and help to relieve stress in the gastrointestinal tract and throughout the body.

What to Use

Take 250 milligrams of chamomile flower oil, 200 milligrams of peppermint leaf oil, and 20 milligrams of English lavender flower oil before or up to 30 minutes after starting every meal. The chamomile should be standardized to 2.5 to 5.5 percent (6.25 to 13.75 milligrams) of apigenin glycosides. The peppermint should supply a minimum of 50 percent (100 milligrams) total menthol. Take the three oils in the form of a combination product for best results.

SUPPLEMENTS FOR SPECIAL CIRCUMSTANCES

Some people may have one or two special circumstances that will require them to use some additional supplements. I will describe the products here, but will discuss the special circumstances in full detail in Chapter 6, "The Step-by-Step Thought Process."

Anti-Anaerobic Bacteria Supplements

Anaerobic bacteria are organisms that live in your gut and feed on sugar. Any time you eat carbohydrates, all of which break down into simple sugars, you feed these bacteria. Your guests then repay you for your trouble with symptoms such as nausea, stomach pain, gas, bloating, burping, and belching.

To determine if you have anaerobic bacteria, see Chapter 6, "Step One: Are You Uncomfortable After Every Meal?" If, after reading the entire section, you determine that your answer to the question posed there is yes, you'll need to add two anti-anaerobic bacteria supplements to your program. The first product should contain a combination of coptis root and rhizome extract, Indian barberry root extract, and berberine sulfate. The second should contain a combination of corydalis yanhusuo tuber *(Corydalis yanhusuo)*, astragalus root *(Astragalus membranaceus)*, tienchi ginseng root *(Panax pseudoginseng)*, zhejiang fritillary bulb *(Fritillaria thunbergii)*, Chinese licorice root *(Glycyrrhiza uralensis)*, gambir leaf and stem *(Uncaria gambir)*, brown's lily bulb *(Lillium brownii)*, bletilla root *(Bletilla striata)*, and cuttlefish shell *(Sepia esculenta)*. These nutrients will work together to promote a healthy mucosal lining as well as a healthy microbial environment in your intestines.

What They Do

The combination of coptis root and rhizome, Indian barberry root, and berberine sulfate supports immune function and encourages the body to purge unwanted compounds. It promotes healthy intestinal microbial balance and detoxification of the liver, gallbladder, and urinary tract. It also helps calm the digestive tract.

The corydalis yanhusuo tuber combination is currently used in more than fifty healing institutions throughout China to promote stomach and duodenal health. It helps to relieve occasional heartburn and acid indigestion, settles an upset stomach, and acts as a local antispasmodic. It also nourishes and protects the mucosal layer of the stomach and duodenum, supporting the health and function of this important protective barrier and maintaining a healthy microbial environment.

What to Use

Take two tablets of the coptis-barberry-berberine combination, each containing at least 400 milligrams of berberine, twenty to thirty minutes before every meal.

Take two 1,500-milligram tablets of the corydalis yanhusuo tuber combination twenty to thirty minutes before every meal.

Peptic Ulcer Disease Supplement

Have you been diagnosed with peptic ulcer disease? There's a relatively new all-natural treatment for it that will completely heal your ulcers. It's called zinc carnosine, and it's composed of one molecule each of zinc and L-carnosine.

Zinc is an essential nutrient. It supports immune function and, important for our purposes, facilitates wound healing. It can be found in beef, pork, seafood, beans, and nuts. L-carnosine is an amino acid that has antioxidant abilities and helps regulate the production of stomach acid.

What It Does

When zinc and L-carnosine are joined together, an unusual nutrient is formed that is water insoluble and heat stable. This nutrient protects the cells of the stomach and encourages their normal metabolism. It performs as an antioxidant, acts as an anti-inflammatory, and inhibits the ulcer-causing bacteria *Helicobacter pylori*. It adheres to ulcers on the stomach wall, protecting them from stomach acid and stimulating their healing. More than twenty studies have been published about this patented nutrient, which has been used in Japan since 1994.

What to Use

Take 75 milligrams of zinc carnosine twice a day, between meals.

The beauty of all-natural medicine is in its availability and lack of side effects. All of the supplements discussed in this chapter are available at your local health food store and online sources. Please see the Essential Supplements section of the Resource List at the back of this book.

In Chapter 5, we will learn about the dietary rules that are a very important part of this protocol. These rules may be the most difficult part of this advice for some of you to follow, but they should be taken seriously. And remember, they are not forever; hopefully, they are just for the time being.

CHAPTER 5

The Big Four
Don't-You-Dare-Break-'Em
Dietary Rules

constipation

ulcers

blood

pain

gas

indigestion

spasms

heartburn

bloating

diarrhea

reflux

GERD

*T*he supplements discussed in Chapter 4 will help to bring health back to your gastrointestinal system. They can't do the job alone, however. For complete recovery from IBS, you need to couple the supplements with dietary changes.

You'll need to make a few lifestyle changes to accomplish the dietary changes recommended in this chapter, but that's all they are—lifestyle changes. Making these changes may seem difficult at first, but there's good reason for them, and if you're reading this book, you're already motivated. In fact, most of the people who ask for my help with IBS are so motivated that if I asked them to go out in their backyards at midnight on the second Tuesday of each month, get down on all fours, and eat crabgrass, they'd do it. I'd have to give them one heck of a reason to do it, of course, but hopefully, the information in this book gives you enough reason to make the dietary changes I suggest. Let's try to avoid the grass stains on your knees.

THE BIG FOUR DIETARY RULES

The following four initial dietary changes are the ones that have given most of the people I've treated for IBS the biggest bang for the effort. Remember, these changes are temporary. If you're lucky, you won't need to make them on a permanent basis. They may initially seem difficult, but trust me, all of my office patients have been able to make them. You'll be able to make them, too.

Big Rule Number One: Avoid Dairy Products

Got milk? Remember those ads with all the celebrities and their milk mustaches? What a great marketing campaign. But guess what the real purpose is for cow's milk. It's food for baby cows. Period! If you're human, it's not intended for you; you shouldn't be drinking it. And if you have IBS or are chronically unwell with any set of gastrointestinal symptoms, you'll find it vital to eliminate dairy products.

I am well aware that this is the most difficult recommendation of mine to follow. It's also the lifestyle change that offers the greatest potential reward. It's that important.

The importance of dairy products in our diets has been drummed into our heads by advertising and marketing since the 1960s, when teachers began tacking posters of the four food groups onto bulletin boards in every classroom in America. Today, we take for granted that milk helps build strong bones. But this is totally untrue. No scientific evidence supports the idea that milk drinkers have stronger bones or more bone mass than people who don't drink milk. Not one study has found this. In addition, no scientific evidence supports the idea that osteoporosis results from not drinking enough milk. If you have ever seen a study that does, please send it to me. Instead, Harvard University has found the opposite. In a twelve-year study beginning in 1976 and following 78,000 women, researchers found that the participants who ate or drank the equivalent of two glasses of milk per day had a 40-percent increased risk of fracture over the participants who consumed less. So much for the benefits of milk.

Let's look at a few other commonsense issues. No other mammal on earth drinks the breast milk of another mammal after it's been weaned off its mother's milk. Humans are the only mammals that do this. The others all drink water. Humans are also the only mammals that consume milk products after infancy. Have you ever seen a bear or giraffe with osteoporosis?

I always suggest to my patients that they eat foods only in the forms nature intended. Milk that has been heated to a very high temperature, which is done during homogenization and pasteurization, is not as nature intended it to be. It lacks anything "live"; all of its enzymes and nutrients have been destroyed or altered. It's a dead food. If we all had cows in our backyards and drank just fresh, raw, unprocessed milk, it would be a different story. It's a far better product than processed milk and doesn't cause as many health problems.

A related issue is lactose intolerance. How many people do you know who claim to be lactose intolerant? In my opinion, almost everyone is lactose intolerant to some degree. When consuming milk, some people experience indigestion, gas, or bloating. Some experience diarrhea or constipation. Some experience all of these symptoms. Because you don't experience any of the symptoms commonly related to lactose intolerance, you don't necessarily not have problems at the chemical and molecular level that might be interfering with your health. Think of it this way: A lack of symptoms isn't what defines health. You're just unaware of the symptoms. And here's why this is a problem.

As infants, humans secrete high amounts of lactase, the enzyme necessary for the proper breakdown of lactose, or milk sugar. Here we go again with those pesky enzymes! The reason for this high secretion of lactase is that infants are intended to subsist on their mother's milk, so their bodies secrete enough of the enzyme to break down the milk's lactose content. After about the age of two, however, lactase secretion substantially declines. Why? Because in humans, birth to age two is the breast-feeding window—that is, most humans finish breast-feeding by the age of two. As a result, after age two, humans have a difficult time digesting milk sugar. Some cultures and ethnic groups have enjoyed a genetic change minimizing the consequences of dairy consumption after age two, but even they have not eliminated them.

Lactose is only one part of the milk molecule. Protein is also found in milk and presents an entirely different problem. Did you know that milk protein is also difficult for the human body to digest? Not because the body lacks sufficient enzymes, but because the protein molecules in milk are held together so tightly, it's difficult for the body to break them apart even with sufficient enzymes. If the milk molecule reaches an area of the gastrointestinal system with subclinical inflammation resulting from a loss of bacterial balance and proper chemistry, it will cross over into the bloodstream, causing the immune system to react and release histamine. A food allergy results. For a detailed discussion of food allergies, see Chapter 7.

Milk is the number-one food allergen found in food allergy testing, because of its protein content, not milk sugar. Histamine release may be responsible for many of your IBS symptoms, as well as other health problems. One easy way to reduce many of your symptoms is to eliminate the histamine release caused by eating milk products. Give up dairy products. Entirely! It's well worth it.

"Give what up?" "Where is milk found?" "Can I still have ice cream?" "How about yogurt?" I get all kinds of questions from patients trying to negotiate to keep their favorite milk products in their diets. Sorry, we have to eliminate all the variables. By milk or dairy products, we mean the following:

❖ All types of milk, including whole, skim, 1 percent, 2 percent, low fat, no fat, Lactaid brand, and acidophilus milk

❖ All types of cheeses, including asadero, Asiago, blue, brick, Brie, Camembert, Cheddar, colby, cottage cheese, cream cheese, Edam, farmer, Gorgonzola, Gouda, Gruyère, Havarti, Jack, Jarlsburg, Limburger, mascarpone, Muenster, Neufchâtel, Parmesan, pecorino, pot, ricotta, Roquefort, Swiss, and Tilsit

❖ Ice cream

❖ Sour cream

❖ Creamy salad dressings, including French, Thousand Island, Roquefort, blue cheese, ranch, and creamy Italian

❖ Yogurt

In addition, you also need to avoid all packaged, canned, bottled, and prepared foods containing cheese, milk, milk solids, milk proteins, milk byproducts, lactose, whey, or casein. To determine if the foods in your refrigerator, freezer, and cupboards contain these ingredients, read their ingredient lists. Don't take anything for granted. If a product has an ingredient list, you must read it. Just because the front of the package says the item is a veggie burger, it's not necessarily made only from vegetables. Just because the label says it's a nondairy creamer, it doesn't necessarily not contain any dairy.

Restaurants present other problems. Mashed potatoes certainly include milk. Salads often have cheese sprinkled on top. Sauces and fancy creations by the chef may contain all kinds of dairy products. In sit-down restaurants, tell your server that you have an allergy to dairy products and ask for help with ordering. Question everything. You should avoid fast food restaurants completely because of the poor quality of the food, but if you must eat in one, just do your best to try to figure out what the different menu items might contain.

Do you like butter? If you do, go ahead and enjoy it. It's a dairy product, but it's almost pure fat. Milk products have three components—sugar (lactose), protein, and fat. Fat causes none of the problems that milk sugar and milk protein do, so you can eat it without suffering any negative consequences.

What about goat's milk? Chemically, goat's milk has no reason to be included in my no-dairy restriction. It has a different molecular structure than cow's milk and shouldn't affect people who are lactose intolerant or have an allergy to cow's milk. But, I recommend avoiding it anyway. First, it has the potential to cause problems for some people, and by not eating it, you eliminate any questions over whether it's a cause of your symptoms. Second, a lot of products that people believe are made from goat's milk are really made from cow's milk with the addition of enzymes. In addition, some goat's-milk products have cow's milk added. I advise staying away from goat's milk until you're completely symptom-free.

Have you noticed how much space I've devoted to dairy products? That's how seriously you should take this information. I remember a patient who, in talking and getting acquainted before beginning our consultation, informed me that he worked as a food scientist for Proctor and Gamble. He also let me know that he knew quite a lot about food. He was a very detail-oriented person who came to his appointments equipped with studies to discuss, and mailed or e-mailed studies to me in between appointments for later discussion.

He began the program as explained in this book, and he made sure we discussed in detail all four of my initial dietary recommendations. But four to six weeks went by, and we didn't see as much progress as I had thought we would. When that happens, I usually ask a lot of questions about the person's diet. What did you eat yesterday? What did you have as snacks? What was in the foods and snacks? I also usually ask the patient to bring any questionable food products to his or her next appointment so that I can look at the packaging myself. We got nowhere.

Finally, this patient admitted to me that he had been eating lunch in the cafeteria at work every day, and he found the mashed potatoes there to be the best he'd ever had. He believed, being the food scientist he was, that if he gave up about 85 percent of his dairy

Clarified Butter

My no-dairy rule calls for the elimination of all dairy products except butter. A handful of times in my career, however, I've seen patients who also couldn't tolerate butter. The reason was extreme lactose intolerance. Though butter is only 1-percent lactose, that was enough to cause problems in these people.

If you follow all of the dietary guidelines in this book and don't seem to get results, consider eliminating butter from your diet. If butter is one of your guilty pleasures and you really miss it, try switching to clarified butter. Clarified butter is lactose-free. You can purchase clarified butter at most health food stores or you can make it on your own.

Clarified butter is butter that has been melted and made clear by having its milk solids separated out and discarded. The milk solids are what contain the protein and lactose. When butter is melted, it separates into a clear golden liquid and a thick liquid that includes the milk solids. As an added benefit, once the milk solids are removed, the remaining butter can be cooked over very high heat without burning.

Clarifying butter is very easy. Cut one stick of butter into small pieces and place the pieces in a heavy saucepan over low heat. When the butter crackles and bubbles, remove the pan from the heat and use a spoon to carefully skim off the fat foam that has risen to the top. Pour or spoon the clear liquid forming the middle layer into a clean container, and discard the thick milky stuff forming the bottom layer. Cover the container with a tightly fitting lid, and refrigerate it for up to several months.

Cheddar Cheese

There is a difference of opinion in the advice you may have heard about which dairy products can or cannot be eaten by people suffering from gastrointestinal problems. Some dietary advice suggests that Cheddar cheese, cottage cheese, blue cheese, yogurt, and any other "fermented" dairy products are suitable to consume. The reason for this is that the fermentation process changes the molecular structure of the components of these products, making them quite different foods than what they began as. This is true, but beware.

My advice is to eliminate *all* dairy products except butter because I have found clinically that most patients still have problems with them. Err on the side of being conservative so that you don't end up with any unintended effects that you cannot account for as you progress through my protocol. Don't risk it.

consumption, he would see an 85-percent improvement in his symptoms. Instead, he saw no improvement.

Dairy is an elimination to be taken seriously. If everyone with IBS would take just one suggestion from this book—to give up all dairy products—two thirds would see an improvement in their health. Avoiding milk usually isn't enough to get rid of all of anyone's symptoms, but most people would at least see a difference.

One last note: Eggs are not dairy products. Many people think of them as such because they're found in the dairy section of grocery stores. However, they come from chickens, not cows (in case you didn't already know that).

Big Rule Number Two: Avoid Gas-Causing Foods

Certain foods in the American diet have become notorious for the gas they cause when consumed. Our bodies have trouble breaking these foods down within a specific period of time, resulting in them spoiling in the gastrointestinal tract and giving off a gas. The main villain in the legume family is an indigestible sugar called raffinose. This is the same sugar found in lesser amounts in cruciferous vegetables (see "Help with Cruciferous Vegetables."). We've all joked about this since we were five years old. Beans cause gas, right? Technically, beans are legumes, and the entire legume family is a prime gas-causing food to avoid when healing from IBS.

All beans should be avoided. This includes navy, kidney, black, red, white, garbanzo, lentil, and soy beans. Peas prepared as a vegetable are okay, but when dried and condensed into a thick soup, such as split pea soup, they become hard to digest. Green beans prepared as a vegetable should also be okay to eat. However, avoid all soy products, including tofu, soy milk, and other products made from the protein portion of the soybean. Soybean oil, a fat found everywhere, seems to be of no concern for most people with IBS. Soy lecithin, an emulsifier of fats and also found in many products, should also not be worried about. Peanuts, often mistakenly considered a nut, are a legume and hard to digest. Tree nuts, such as macadamias, almonds, cashews, and walnuts, are fine to consume.

Fruit is a problem for many people when it's combined with other foods. Therefore, I recommend following the old food-combining rule that says to eat fruit only before a meal or all by itself. Fruit is very easily digested and released from the stomach quickly for rapid absorption in the small intestine. However, when it's mixed with other foods or eaten after a meal, it spoils while waiting for the other foods in the stomach to be digested. A common question concerns tomatoes, though they are a fruit, consider them a vegetable when it comes to this rule. Please note that problems with gas caused by the spoilage of fruit waiting to be digested are different from fructose intolerance, which we'll discuss in Chapter 6.

But, Where Do I Get My Calcium?

This is a common question from women. Worried about their bone health, they fear that the no-dairy rule found in this program will cause them harm. I like to attempt to calm those fears by pointing out something that makes sense for everyone.

All the women who ask this question knew another woman, possibly their mother, grandmother, aunt, or friend, who discussed her diagnosis of osteoporosis. Simply walking down the street, they may have seen women with a dowager's hump, which is a hump that appears in older women at the base of the neck (top of the shoulders) and is a sign of advanced bone loss.

The one sure thing all these women had in common was that they ate all the dairy products they ever wanted during the course of their life. So, what happened?

This proves a point: The use of dairy products is not the way to prevent osteoporosis. Remember my story about how all other animals simply drink water.

As usual with health issues, this story is really not this simple. Calcium metabolism and bone health are not dependent only on eating *absorbable* forms of calcium (mostly from plant material), but also on hormone balance and exercise. Exercise is up to the individual, and hormone balance is a complex issue all its own. One thing is for certain: Women should have no fears about restricting their dairy intake for the time frame it takes to conquer their gastrointestinal symptoms—or forever.

Lactaid, Acidophilus Milk, and Activia Yogurt

As if the readers of this book need any additional proof of the importance of digestive enzymes or probiotics, let's take a look at what traditional food companies have recently begun to produce.

Lactaid

Based on the well-known fact that many people have trouble digesting the lactose (a form of sugar) in dairy products, the product Lactaid was created. Though a logical attempt, the product fails in two ways. First, the digestive enzyme that is added to the milk is very weak and may not help with the complete digestion of the milk sugar, leaving many consumers with all or most of their digestive discomfort.

Second, as I have discussed in this section, the protein portion of the dairy product may be as much of a villain as the lactose portion. Lactaid does not address this problem at all and will be completely ineffective for the people who have a problem with the protein part of dairy.

Acidophilus Milk

With public awareness growing about the importance of probiotics, some milk producers are seeing an opportunity to capitalize on the media attention by putting acidophilus into their milk. Wait! Doesn't placing probiotics in milk create yogurt?

(continued on page 67)

Some people also have problems with cruciferous vegetables. These vegetables aren't known as gas-causing foods for the general public. They just cause gas in people with imbalanced gastrointestinal systems. Once a person's gastrointestinal system is balanced and functioning efficiently again, these foods should no longer cause any problems. The cruciferous vegetables include:

❖ Arugula

❖ Bok choy

❖ Broccoli

❖ Brussels sprouts

❖ Cabbage

❖ Cauliflower

❖ Chinese cabbage

❖ Collard greens

❖ Daikon

❖ Kale

❖ Kohlrabi

❖ Mustard greens

❖ Radishes

❖ Rutabaga

❖ Turnips

❖ Watercress

Many people also have problems consuming other foods that don't seem to cause trouble for anyone else.

If you do, stay away from these foods. If most foods seem to cause you discomfort, do your best to stay away from as many as possible, but remember that you do need to eat something. Consider yourself as being in a transition. You are going from where you are today when it comes to what you believe you can or cannot eat to a time when you will be far more comfortable and can eat a wider variety of foods. How long this takes is different for everyone. You must have the confidence to test foods as you progress through the protocol. Taking digestive enzymes might make all the difference in the world, and some of the foods you think will cause you trouble might not anymore.

When your gastrointestinal system is balanced and healthy again, you'll be able to slowly add more foods back into your diet. Even before this time, you may find foods along the way that you thought you couldn't tolerate but now can.

Vegetarians, especially, may have problems avoiding gas-causing foods. If you're a vegetarian, the legume family probably makes up a large percentage of your daily food intake because of the protein contained in them. If you're accustomed to eating a lot of legumes and gas and bloating are not among your symptoms, you can ignore this rule. However, if gas and bloating are problems for you, see if you can cut back on your legume intake just a bit for a short period of time. The additional digestive enzymes I recommend for everyone in Chapter 4 will

(continued from page 66)

Well, it should. The strains of acidophilus used in acidophilus milk are weak and will "ferment" the milk only a small degree. No yogurt here. This also means the milk will not be effective at reestablishing the beneficial bacteria balances to any worthwhile degree.

Activia Yogurt

A more recent addition to the dairy section, Activia yogurt is one of the more well-thought-out products. The manufacturer has decided to use a very specific strain of probiotic called *Bifidus regularis*. Each serving of Activia has billions of organisms, and this product may very well help some patients with gastrointestinal complaints.

But, beware. Yes, our knowledge of probiotics suggests that this product could be helpful. It sounds logical. The problem is that although the little critters in the product might be great for you, the lactose and the protein contents may not. Yogurt has both of those, and your discomfort may actually increase with use of this product.

Balance your beneficial bacteria levels by using good probiotic supplements, such as those discussed in the Essential Supplements section of the Resource List at the back of this book.

also assist your body in digesting these foods and will help to reduce the symptoms associated with them. Otherwise, if you remain a vegetarian, you may just have to put up with some gas and bloating.

Can't I Have Just a Little Dairy?

I get this question all the time. Patients continually try to negotiate their favorite foods into this plan. Some cheat, and some make what they think is an intellectual, logical decision about the amount of dairy they are willing to give up.

Many years ago, I came across a patient who really woke me up regarding the importance of following the rules in this book. These rules must be followed 100 percent. No ifs, ands or buts.

As you probably have noticed, the dietary villains I mention in this book are not discussed with the thought that perhaps you should cut back on them and see what happens. My advice is to completely cut them out of your diet.

A female patient came to me with diarrhea and bowel movements ten to fifteen times each day. (If you don't suffer from diarrhea, the point of this story should still be taken seriously). We made it about eight to ten weeks into my treatment plan and she was not getting any better. I asked her my usual laundry list of questions while trying to figure out what we might be missing, and she finally admitted what she called her "logical decision" about the dairy she was eating.

(continued on page 69)

Big Rule Number Three: Do Not Drink Liquids During or Directly After Meals

Drinking enough water every day is certainly very important. I always tell my patients to make pure water their main drink and to shoot for a daily intake of eight large glasses. However, while on my program to heal IBS, you shouldn't drink anything—water included—during meals or for an hour afterward.

As food travels through the body, its first stop is the stomach. In the stomach, if the food contains protein, and sometimes even if it doesn't, it initiates the secretion of hydrochloric acid. As we discussed in Chapter 3, hydrochloric acid is the digestive enzyme that begins the breakdown of proteins. If you add liquid to the mix, you dilute the strength of the hydrochloric acid and diminish its ability to break down the proteins within a certain amount of time. Diluted hydrochloric acid is about as effective at breaking down protein as a thimbleful of ammonia in a swimming pool's worth of water is at cleaning a kitchen floor. As we have also discussed, gas and bloating are the result of not breaking down food within a certain amount of time.

Another reason not to drink during meals or for an hour afterward is heartburn. Food in the stomach should be chewed and soft, not watery. If you add too much liquid, you create a soup. When hydrochloric acid is added to the mix, it becomes an acidic soup. Because of its consistency, this acidic soup may splash back up into the esophagus, burning the tissue and causing what we know as heartburn. It doesn't matter if you secrete too much or too little hydrochloric acid. Any amount will create an acidic soup. This explains why so many people take antacids in the belief that they produce too much acid. Most people don't. They just have an acidic soup. It also explains why so many people feel discomfort when lying in bed. With the body in that position, it's even easier for the acidic soup to splash up into the esophagus.

When you drink between meals, make water your drink of choice. Coffee and tea, especially unsweetened, are fine if not taken in excess. Fruit juices, however, should be limited. Have you ever watched those old movies with the crazy-looking scientists pouring chemicals into glass beakers in dark, dingy basements? All of a sudden the liquid starts to bubble up and flow out of the beaker. This can happen in your stomach. It's usually due to two or more incompatible liquids or foods being mixed together. Water is neutral, so it plays well with all other liquids, which is why it's always the best drink option.

What about soup? Good question. Soup is a liquid that often also contains solid food. Let's simplify the problem by saying that soup, like fruit, should be eaten either by itself or at the very beginning of a meal.

If you're afraid that you won't have enough time in the day to drink your quota of water, think again. Granted,

(continued from page 68)

She hated black coffee. She heard my story about not using cream and how a nondairy creamer was not nondairy. But since she had some in her cupboard, she decided to use it. Since a nondairy creamer is mostly chemicals, she thought, how much dairy product could possibly be in the one teaspoon she was putting into each of the two cups of coffee she drank each morning?

She gave up the practice, and two weeks later, she was having bowel movements just twice a day and they were solid and formed. It was that fast! What this illustrates is that I never know, nor do my patients ever know, how sensitive they may be to any of the dietary villains I try to identify for them. Bottom line: These rules need to be followed 100 percent of the time. Don't cheat!

Do You Like Spicy Food?

Surprisingly to me, since I don't tend to season my food with much but salt and very little pepper, I have found that many of my patients love spicy foods or lots of pepper. It may be helpful to mention that when patients seem not to be getting well, I ask them what spices they use.

I can safely say that if you love spicy foods—and especially hot spices like cayenne (red pepper), cumin, curry, mustard, wasabi, garlic, or hot peppers—you may find that they may be part of what's causing your discomfort and symptoms. Even black pepper can be irritating enough to cause problems. The best solution? Eat a bland diet and forgo the spices until you get a handle on why you have your symptoms.

Also, check all spice blends for the inclusion of monosodium glutamate (MSG), and also look for it in the ingredient list of any packaged foods you may eat, because it is known to cause gastrointestinal discomfort and other symptoms.

most people drink the majority of their day's water right before, during, and after their meals. According to rule number three, you're restricted from drinking water for a total of about four or five hours a day. Take away another eight hours for sleep, and you're left with eleven to twelve hours a day to get in your eight glasses. I know this is a lifestyle change, but it's one that's well worth it. In addition, like the other rules, this one may also be temporary. Once balance is restored to your gastrointestinal system, you may find that you're once again able to tolerate some liquids during your meals.

Big Rule Number Four:
Do Not Take Your Regular Vitamin, Mineral, or Herbal Supplements

"What?" I hear you saying. "I thought those were good for me!" Your regular vitamin, mineral, and herbal supplements might be excellent products, and they might do you a lot of good under normal circumstances, but for a short period of time, you'll be better off not taking them. The reason for stopping these products is to temporarily remove any potential confounding variables from the equation.

Please don't assume you're buying high-quality products just because you're getting them from a trusted health food store or a friend who sells a well-known multi-level line of health supplements. And if they are high quality, they could still be contributing to your problem. Eliminating them for a short period of time (about four to eight weeks) might provide valuable clues.

DON'T ASK ME WHAT YOU SHOULD EAT

My patients ask me all the time, "Just tell me what to eat."

My answer: "No!"

The request usually arises for one of a couple of different reasons. My typical IBS patients know that certain foods bother them, and they do their best to try to figure out which foods these are. But they can't figure it out completely no matter what they do, and they think that I should know. I don't know, however, because IBS is such a complex condition and every patient has his or her own biochemical individuality. The foods that are the villains are different for everybody.

Other patients, after eliminating the foods recommended in this chapter as well as some or all of the other food groups mentioned in Chapter 6, despair that they have nothing left to eat, so plead with me to give them some options. Don't give up; don't feel frustrated. Remember, this program is a process. Following the dietary restrictions in this chapter may be enough for you; you may never have to add the ones in Chapter 6. The majority of my patients don't, because we eliminate their symptoms using just the Big Four Don't-You-*Dare*-Break-'Em Dietary Rules.

People are creatures of habit. You may simply need to think about your food choices a bit more instead of just taking them for granted. Even if you have to follow every dietary restriction in this book, you'll still have food choices left—fresh beef, pork,

Help with Cruciferous Vegetables

If you continue to have problems with the cruciferous family of vegetables even after healing your gastrointestinal system, you can try taking a digestive enzyme called Aspergillus oryzae, derived from a fungus and containing the enzymes amylase, protease, lipase and cellulase.

Cruciferous vegetables cause a problem for many people because despite their healthy profile, they have a bad reputation as gas producers due to their content of an indigestible sugar called raffinose. (As previously mentioned, even larger amounts of raffinose are found in beans, which are notorious for inducing flatulence.) Methane-producing bacteria in the colon feed on raffinose and release gas in the process. There's nothing you can do to broccoli and the other crucifers to cut down on the gas they induce. The extent to which your body produces gas depends on the types of bacteria in your colon that break down foods for digestion, and restoring the beneficial bacteria levels may well lead to a reduction in the amount of gas you produce when eating cruciferous vegetables.

poultry, seafood, eggs, nuts, rice, white potatoes, and the allowed vegetables. Anyone can live on these choices.

In this chapter, we discussed the four lifestyle changes everyone with IBS should adopt. You may wish you didn't have to adopt them, but you really should. These dietary changes will eliminate the variables that seem to cause the majority of symptoms in my office patients with IBS. Dairy products historically are a problem for people with gastrointestinal symptoms, so we eliminate them first. We eliminate gas-causing foods because they may mask other reasons for the gas. Not eating fruit with other foods and not drinking liquids during or for one hour after meals gives digestion a little assistance and helps to eliminate not only gas, but also heartburn, reflux, and GERD. Discontinuing any supplements you might be taking from other sources rounds out our elimination of as many variables as possible. All of these eliminations are intended to be temporary, and hopefully will help identify the real villains in your diet.

In the next chapter, we will learn about a very important approach to working your way through this complex and at times confusing path to healthier gastrointestinal function. I have a step-by-step thought process that is important for all patients to understand, as it will help you make the right decision at the different points in your treatment program.

CHAPTER 6

The Step-by-Step Thought Process

constipation

ulcers

blood

pain

gas

indigestion

spasms

heartburn

bloating

diarrhea

reflux

GERD

In previous chapters, we discussed my Big Four Don't-You-*Dare*-Break-'Em Dietary Rules and the supplements I recommend. But how do you implement all of this information?

THE STEP-BY-STEP PROCESS

The step-by-step thought process I use with this program is just as important as—and possibly even more important than—everything else we've discussed thus far. Without an understanding of it, you might find yourself heading toward failure. That's because there may be times, as you're working your way through the program, that you will find a situation come up that makes no sense. It's at that time that you'll need to rely on the thought process. The thought process covers almost all the situations that may come up, and in general, it explains what to do if one or possibly two stubborn symptoms persist. It will help you to

Case History: Walter

Walter was an 86-year-old World War II vet. He came to my office in diapers. This almost brought tears to my eyes, as here was the toughest of the tough, someone who had been through the unimaginable and survived. And the last years of his life were reduced to this. He was angry.

Walter complained of diarrhea and an urgency that he was unable to control and required diapers to prevent accidents. He had a bowel movement about ten times a day, not counting the accidents. He began my protocol for irritable bowel syndrome.

We saw minimal success and began to follow the Step-by-Step Thought Process outlined in this chapter. The stool testing was of little help, as was the elimination of fructose and gluten. Still, we didn't see much success. Walter was about as frustrated as any patient I had ever seen.

One day, he showed up unexpectedly at my office and asked to see me. He told me he had decided to ask his gastroenterologist to remove part of his intestines and provide him with a colostomy bag. He was tired of the pain, inconvenience, and

(continued on page 76)

formulate a specific plan to follow regarding the use of the supplements, the beginning dietary eliminations, the additional dietary eliminations, and the laboratory testing.

The stubborn symptoms that usually remain are gas and diarrhea. However, as is true of IBS in general, the stubborn symptoms you experience may be different. No matter what symptoms you find persisting in your individual case, the step-by-step thought process will guide you in tackling them. I use this thought process with all of my office patients who have stubborn symptoms, and I always find the answer to conquering those symptoms within its steps.

If you find yourself confronted with a confusing situation or one or two symptoms that just won't resolve, work through the following steps in order.

Step One: Are You Uncomfortable After Every Meal?

Before we even get started, I ask each of my office patients a simple question: Do you have gas and/or bloating and/or burping/belching and/or stomach discomfort of any kind associated with your upper gastrointestinal system (belly button and up) that occurs immediately to forty-five minutes after you sit down to eat every meal? Some people find these symptoms setting in before they even get up from the table. If you answer yes to this question, you have an anaerobic-bacteria problem that must be eliminated before you can begin to feel better.

Please note that the key word in this question is "every." You will be complaining of a noticeable increase in symptoms after beginning to eat every meal. You will not have to think about the question before answering it. You will have no doubt whether or not your symptoms increase. Note that we're not talking about gas that

(continued from page 75)

loss of quality of life. He rationalized this because he figured he had very few years left and the colostomy bag would make those few remaining years more tolerable.

I begged him to reconsider, as we had not yet taken one of the most important steps in my protocol—the food allergy test. He said he had no more money left to devote to figuring this out. As his insurance had not covered my protocol, I told him I would contact the insurance company to fight for coverage. Finally, the insurance company consented.

The allergy test revealed foods that he should stay away from, and within two weeks he started to see positive changes that began to give him hope. In less than a month, his bowel movements were solid and reduced to two or three per day.

you may have all day long or at different times of the day. We're not talking about nausea that you may have after some meals. These are intermittent symptoms. We're also not talking about the need to have a bowel movement after eating every meal.

If your answer to this question is no, or if you're unsure of your answer, you do not have an anaerobic-bacteria problem. Please move on to Step Two.

So, what are anaerobic bacteria? They are organisms that live on sugar, not oxygen. Any time you eat something that contains carbohydrates, these organisms love it and repay you for your kindness with discomfort, nausea, pain, gas and/or bloating, burping/belching, or other symptoms usually associated with your upper gastrointestinal system. All carbohydrates, whether simple or complex carbohydrates and including fruits, vegetables, grains, rice, potatoes—even lettuce--break down into the same sugar contained in candy bars. It's called glucose. If you eat the average American diet—high in carbohydrates and full of sweets—you're in trouble.

Anaerobic bacteria live in the first foot or so of the small intestine, the perfect spot to wait for carbohydrates (sugar) to be released from the stomach. As soon as any stomach content is released or simply seeps out of the stomach, they begin to feed and become more active. It's this activity that causes the increased symptoms after every meal. If you're unsure whether you have anaerobic bacteria, try eating only protein and fat for one or two meals. For example, eat just a plain beef patty, a plain chicken breast, or tuna right out of the can. These foods have no carbs, and you shouldn't experience any increase in symptoms.

If you believe you have anaerobic bacteria, begin taking the essential supplements to reestablish bacterial balance (see Chapter Four) and the essential supplements to improve digestion and restore pH (see Chapter Four). However, do not take the essential supplements to feed the tissue and restore cChemistry. Instead, take the anti-anaerobic bacteria supplements (see Chapter Four), which contain herbs that are antimicrobial and will eliminate the anaerobic bacteria from your upper gastrointestinal tract. Also, implement the dietary restrictions explained in Chapter 5.

After taking the anti-anaerobic bacteria supplements for one month, you'll need to make your first judgment call. Are you feeling better? If your answer is yes, move on to Step Two. But what if you're not feeling better? Most people need to take the anti-anaerobic bacteria supplements for one month, but a small percentage of people need to take them for another month. About 1 to 2 percent of people need to take them for longer periods. My recommendation is to continue taking the anti-anaerobic bacteria supplements for one more month, to make sure you get rid of your anaerobic-bacteria population.

If you prefer a quicker and more powerful remedy for anaerobic bacteria than the herbal supplements I recommend, you can try a prescription antibiotic called Flagyl. Flagyl is faster acting (it works in seven to ten days, compared to one month for the herbs), but it will damage your population of good bacteria much more than the herbs will. Prescription antibiotics also have detrimental effects on the liver, which natural herbs do not.

Step Two: Begin the Essential Supplement Program

If you have decided that you don't have an anaerobic-bacteria problem, begin to take all the essential supplements described in Chapter 4 and implement the dietary restrictions explained in Chapter 5.

If you had an anaerobic-bacteria problem and either successfully treated it or decided to move on to Step Two anyway, begin taking all the essential supplements described in Chapter 4 by adding those to feed the tissue and restore chemistry (see Chapter Four).

Step Three: Whoa! What's That Smell?

If, within a day or two of beginning to take all the essential supplements in Step Two, you begin to experience additional gas and/or bloating, you will need to have a stool test (see the Laboratory Tests section in the Resource List). Having increased gas and/or bloating right after starting to take FOS is a clinical indicator that you have something living inside you that needs to be identified and then eliminated.

As explained in Chapter 4, FOS is a sugar that humans can't metabolize. In other words, we could eat it all day, and it would just pass out of our bodies. In my protocol, we use it to feed the good bacteria in the gastrointestinal system. It helps to provide an environment that's conducive for the reproduction of this healthful population.

However, if you have organisms living inside you that shouldn't be there, they will also eat this sugar, and when they do, they will become more active and give off a gas as a metabolic byproduct. Once again, you'll have no doubt whether or not you're experiencing additional gas and/or bloating. In fact, it could be so obvious that your family will ask you to move out of the house! The good news is that it will last for only a day or two. So, discontinue taking the FOS.

In addition, arrange for a stool test to identify what's living inside you that shouldn't be there. Test kits are available from a number of laboratories around the country (see the Laboratory Tests section in the Resource List at the back of this book). Follow the directions discussed there to take the test, interpret the results, and treat the problems it reveals, then take a retest to make sure you've resolved the issues. Do not discontinue taking the essential supplements to reestablish bacterial balance or the essential supplements to improve digestion and restore pH.

Gas and/or Bloating

Let's clear up a common point of confusion: You can't become bloated without having gas. I have had patients tell me that they become bloated but they don't have any gas. This is impossible. (Remember, we're not talking about female menstrual bloating from water gain or good old-fashioned weight gain.) What these people mean is they become bloated but they don't burp it up this way or pass it out the other way. So, if you experience additional gas *and/or* bloating within the first day or two of taking FOS, you need a lab test.

Step Four: Let's Make Sure

If you have survived the first day or two without your family asking you to move out—that is, you didn't experience additional gas and/or bloating, or if you did, you had a stool test performed and resolved the problem it revealed—but you still have symptoms such as gas and/or bloating and/or stomach discomfort, you need to double-check that you're following the Big Four Don't-You-*Dare*-Break-'Em Dietary Rules.

Are you avoiding dairy products? Remember, you need to completely cut out dairy products. If you just eliminate most dairy products, you might not see any improvement at all. Read the discussion of this rule again (see Chapter 5), and check all labels for milk, cheese, lactose, whey, and casein. Make sure you're not mistakenly eating anything that contains dairy because you're assuming it doesn't.

In addition to avoiding dairy products, are you also avoiding gas-causing foods? Are you drinking primarily water, and drinking it just between meals, not during meals or within one hour afterwards? Have you stopped taking your non-program supplements? For discussions of these rules, see Chapter 5.

Step Five: The No-Fructose Rule

If you can honestly say that you're completely avoiding dairy products and following the other three Don't-You-*Dare*-Break-'Em Dietary Rules but you still have symptoms, you need to begin avoiding fructose. Fructose is contained in all fruits; natural sweeteners such as sugar, honey, molasses, and maple syrup; corn and corn products such as corn syrup and high-fructose corn syrup; and sweet vegetables such as beets, carrots, eggplant, peas, onions, tomatoes, sweet potatoes, turnips, and winter squash (acorn, buttercup, calabaza, delicate, Hubbard, spaghetti, sweet dumpling and turban). If fructose is your problem, you should see a reduction in your symptoms within a week or so.

Since fructose is found in sugar, you will need to make sure you eliminate all foods with added sugar. To do this, you need to read ingredient lists, which you're doing anyway to make sure you're not consuming any dairy products. But don't confuse a product's ingredient list with its "Nutrition Facts" label. This label describes the product's serving size, total servings per container, and total fat, cholesterol, sodium, total carbohydrate, sugar, and protein content, along with vitamin and mineral content. The sugar mentioned here is not what concerns us. We're talking about added sugar, not the naturally occurring sugars that come from the carbohydrates in food. Yes, all carbohydrates break down into sugar, but again, that's not the sugar with which we're concerned in this step.

Now, why are we so concerned with fructose? Dietary fructose intolerance is the inability to absorb fructose because of a lack of the mucosal enzymes necessary for their digestion. This inability to absorb fructose usually causes gas and/or bloating or diarrhea. It may also cause other symptoms. Once the tissue lining the inside of your gastrointestinal tract is healthy again, you may regain the ability to absorb fructose without symptoms. How long that takes is different for different people. Some people never regain the ability.

A small percentage of people may have a condition called hereditary fructose intolerance, which is different from dietary fructose intolerance. Hereditary fructose intolerance is a genetically caused lack of production of the enzyme l-phosphofructaldolase. This enzyme is not related to the digestion of food, but plays a role in a far more complex chemical process involving fructose. A lack of this enzyme produces more serious symptoms than gastrointestinal problems, including hypoglycemia and liver damage.

Step Six: The No-Gluten Rule

If eliminating fructose from the diet doesn't seem to do the trick, the next thing to try is eliminating gluten. Gluten is contained in foods such as wheat, oats, barley, and rye. This is also a 100-percent elimination, as there will be no room for allowing any in your diet. If a food from a package, bottle, can, box, or frozen convenience food has an ingredient list, read it before you begin eating.

Wheat is made into flour and may be called white flour, whole wheat flour, bleached flour, or unbleached flour on an ingredient list. Breads, cookies, cakes, crackers, bagels, and pasta are some foods that contain wheat. You will also find wheat added to other convenience or frozen foods. If the food is breaded, it's breaded with wheat. Gluten is also found on dried fruits, as they are coated with flour to prevent sticking. Certain sauces and condiments may contain modified food starch, another gluten product.

Oatmeal contains oats, as does granola. Many breakfast bars and protein bars also contain oats.

Barley is found as a grain added to vegetable and other soups, and is also made into regular or white vinegar. As a substitute for white vinegar, use apple cider vinegar, balsamic vinegar or rice vinegar. If you find the word "malt" in an ingredient list, avoid the product, as malt also comes from barley.

Staying away from rye is very easy, as you will almost always find it only in rye bread, which is made from wheat flour with rye flour added.

There are three different problems associated with eating gluten: gluten intolerance, gluten allergy, and celiac disease. Gluten intolerance is when the body is unable to digest or tolerate gluten. The chemistry and consequences of eating gluten-containing foods happen entirely within the digestive tract.

In a gluten allergy, the body becomes allergic to gluten when the gluten-containing foods improperly pass through unhealthy tissue of the digestive tract and enter the bloodstream. Once the food is in the bloodstream, the immune system is called upon to process the food's molecules because they're not supposed to be there. (Please see the discussion of histamine and leaky gut syndrome in Chapter 7.) The immune system creates an antibody and specific chemistry (an immune reaction). This process happens entirely within the bloodstream, yet it has gastrointestinal consequences.

Celiac disease, also called celiac sprue, is an inflammatory condition of the small intestine caused by the ingestion of gluten-containing foods by individuals with a certain type of genetic makeup. The illness most commonly develops around the age of two, after these foods have been introduced into the diet, and in early adult life, between the ages of twenty and forty. However, it can begin at any time in life. In susceptible individuals, the gluten triggers an inflammatory reaction in the small bowel that results in a wearing away of the villi, the tiny fingerlike projections that line the intestines and increase the surface area available for absorbing nutrients. In severe celiac disease, the symptoms may include diarrhea, weakness, and weight loss. In some cases, the primary symptom is anemia-related fatigue, with no symptoms referable to the gastrointestinal tract. In these latter cases, the disease may be limited to the proximal small bowel, where iron is normally absorbed, with the remainder of the bowel in an adequately healthy condition to still properly absorb fluids and the nutrients other than iron. The only solution for a gluten intolerance, gluten allergy, or celiac disease is the elimination of gluten from the diet.

The same as for fructose, once the tissue lining the inside of your gastrointestinal tract is healthy again, non-celiac patients may regain the ability to absorb gluten without symptoms. Again, the length of time it will take to reach that point is different for different people, and some people may never regain the ability.

Step Seven: The Food Allergy Test

If you have done everything recommended in Steps One through Six, and you have done them in the order suggested, but you are still experiencing symptoms, you need to arrange for a food allergy test to be done using your blood. Eighty-eight foods will be tested, and you'll learn exactly what you should no longer eat.

Test kits are available from a number of laboratories around the

Alternatives to Gluten-Containing Foods

What am I going to eat? This is another frequently asked question, especially by people who need to stop eating all gluten-containing foods. A sigh of relief sometimes escapes them—although not all the time—when they learn that there are alternative grains they can use to replace the bread they're used to eating, as well as other grains for baking and use in recipes.

Spelt wheat bread can be found at most major health food stores, and although it contains a small amount of gluten, it usually causes no problems. A number of different bakeries offer spelt breads and not all may appeal to your taste buds, but try a few different kinds until you find one you like. The best ones are almost identical to whole wheat bread in taste, texture, and appearance. Rice breads can also be found in health food stores, but they are not usually as tasty.

Alternative grains are also used for gluten-free and dairy-free cookies. In addition, gluten-free pancake mixes and pasta are made from spelt, rice, and corn.

Look for any products that say "gluten free," as there are more and more people who need to or are electing to become gluten-free and many foods are being produced to fill this marketplace.

country (see the Laboratory Tests section in the Resource List at the back of this book). Follow the directions in this section to take the test and to interpret the results.

Step Eight: What If Nothing Has Worked Yet?

If you still have some symptoms and you did not submit a stool sample in Step Three because you really didn't have additional gas and/or bloating when you first began taking all the supplements, arrange for a stool test to be done now to see whether or not something may have been missed. Another option would be to have a parasite test to see if that may be the problem. I've had to go this far in the process with only a handful of office patients. Your chances of reaching this point are extremely slim.

Test kits are available from a number of laboratories around the country (see the Laboratory Tests section in the Resource List at the back of this book). Follow the directions in this section to take the test, interpret the results, and treat the problem it reveals. When you've finished the protocol, take a retest to make sure you've resolved the issues.

THE CONCEPT OF THE PROCESS OF ELIMINATION

One of the reasons IBS and other gastrointestinal problems are so hard for conventional medicine to conquer is that they're extremely complex and have many variables. Everybody has a unique chemistry, and the reason for the existence of any given symptom can be different for everybody.

My program is based on the process of elimination. The process of elimination helps us to solve the seemingly unsolvable. We use it not only to learn things but to show us what's unnecessary and shouldn't be focused on. It's an entirely different thought process from what most conventional medical doctors use.

Fructose or Gluten?

A judgment call that may be valuable to make involves the no-fructose and no-gluten rules. Although I listed the no-fructose rule first, it may be more effective for you to eliminate all gluten-containing foods first.

The way to determine which rule to institute first is to review which foods have to be eliminated from each food group and then to make a judgment call about which food group contributes more foods to your diet. If you find you eat more gluten than fructose containing foods, eliminate the gluten containing foods first. If you can't decide, just begin with the fructose containing foods.

Research Your Medications' Side Effects

Every medication has side effects. Many of the common medications have gastrointestinal side effects. If you are working your way through the first seven steps of this process and you're still saddled with a symptom or two, you can at any time read the insert that comes with your prescription medication. You know—the large, folded paper the pharmacist staples to the bag that no one reads. You don't have to read the whole thing; just scan it for the two sections labeled "Warnings" and "Adverse Reactions." These two sections will tell you whether or not the medication has possible side effects associated with the gastrointestinal system.

If your medication does have gastrointestinal side effects, you have two choices: (1) Discuss with your doctor the possibility of switching to another medication that will accomplish the same thing but without as many gastrointestinal side effects, or (2) accept that you may have to live with the symptoms. If you choose to do the latter, at least you'll know that your medication may be responsible for your symptoms. If you opt for the first choice, don't go off the medication without your physician's approval.

The purpose of the Big Four Don't-You-*Dare*-Break-'Em Dietary Rules is to remove a number of variables right at the beginning of the program. Right off the bat, you're eliminating four of the major culprits in IBS—dairy products, gas-causing foods, dilution of hydrochloric acid and other digestive enzymes, and nutritional supplements that may be contributing to your symptoms. You then sit back and watch what happens.

If you're lucky, you improve quickly, and you proceed through the three-month program without a hitch. But what if you don't improve?

What if you begin to take the essential supplements, and some or all of your symptoms increase? Now remember, we know what causes an increase in gas or bloating (see Step Three of the Step-by-Step Thought Process). What we're talking about here are other symptoms. So, we may have to back up a little bit. Eliminate all the essential supplements I've suggested you take, wait until the increased symptoms return to where they were before you started the program, and reintroduce the supplements, but one at a time. When your symptoms begin to worsen again, you'll know which supplement is the culprit. If your symptoms don't improve when you go off the supplements, you will know it's not the supplements, but something else, causing the problem. Take a look at the six possible reasons described below.

What if you were going along swimmingly, everything was improving, and you were very pleased, and then suddenly, out of the blue, one or two of your symptoms returned? I've seen this happen time and again with my office patients. It's called backsliding, and it's usually due to one of the following six reasons:

❖ *You haven't yet begun to completely follow all of the Big Four Don't-You-Dare-Break-'Em Dietary Rules, which are all eliminations.* You may initially have seen a positive response with your partial elimination of the restricted foods, but it has caught up with you now, and you need to start taking the rules more seriously.

❖ *You've begun eating new foods that are causing you new problems.* Because of the changes you've had to make in your diet, you've become frustrated with your food choices. In a search for more variety, you've begun to experiment with additional foods that you aren't used to eating. Eliminate all the new foods you've added to your diet and see if the pesky symptoms go away again. If they do, add the new foods back one at a time until your symptoms return, and you'll know which of the new foods is the culprit.

❖ *After a period of time without any symptoms, you've begun to reintroduce some of the foods you've been restricted from eating.* The first time you tried one of these foods, you may not have had a negative reaction. So, you tried it again a few days later, or you tried another restricted food, and again you had no negative reaction. Because these initial attempts were successful and you were happy to have one or more of your favorite foods back, you continued dabbling, being careful to space out your meals or limit your amounts.

The Step-by-Step Thought Process

1. *Are You Uncomfortable After Every Meal?* The first question you must ask yourself before you start.

2. *Begin the Essential Supplement Program.* The must-have, used-by-everybody supplements.

3. *Whoa! What's That Smell?* The clinical indicator that suggests your first lab test.

4. *Step Four: Let's Make Sure.* A double-check to make sure you're on the right track.

5. *The No-Fructose Rule.* The first additional dietary elimination.

6. *The No-Gluten Rule.* The second additional dietary elimination.

7. *The Food allergy Test.* Further dietary eliminations based on science.

8. *What If Nothing Has Worked Yet?* Don't worry too much about this one, since very few people ever get this far.

Artificial Sweeteners

One of my perspectives about maintaining your health centers around eating only natural foods. A good rule of thumb: If man created, processed, or altered the food in any way, the body won't understand it and there will be consequences from eating it. Artificial sweeteners obviously fall into this category. They should be avoided at all costs.

NutraSweet

NutraSweet is formulated from three components—methyl alcohol (methanol) and two amino acids called phenylalanine and aspartic acid.

Manufacturer's Defense. The manufacturer's convoluted defense of the product is that the two amino acids are found naturally in the proteins we eat every day, and that methanol is found naturally in many common foods such as apples. Both statements are true.

The Reality. In nature, the twenty-eight amino acids occur in various combinations and are found in minute quantities. The body carefully regulates the blood and the brain levels of the amino acids for a reason. When found in nature, the amino acids are generally grouped together, which limits the absorption of any single amino acid into your cells. The main problem with NutraSweet is that it contains phenylalanine and aspartic acid as isolated amino acids—that is, they're not limited by the presence of other amino acids and they're present in much higher levels than what are normally found in the proteins we eat. The highly concentrated doses of phenylalanine and aspartic acid found in this artificial sweetener increase their blood and brain concentrations. Independent studies have shown that an increased level of either amino acid is toxic to the brain.

Even more harmful to the human brain is methanol, because at temperatures higher than 86 degrees Fahrenheit, it converts first to formaldehyde and then to a more deadly compound called formic acid. A safe level of exposure has never been established for formaldehyde. Although the manufacturer says that even apples, alcoholic beverages, and other foods contain methanol, what it doesn't mention is that nature always combines methanol with ethanol. Ethanol cancels out methanol's toxicity, except in cases of excessive alcohol ingestion. Methanol is what creates the long-lasting neurological symptoms in alcoholics. Because methanol is a very powerful neurotoxin, the FDA carefully controls it by allowing only minute quantities in food, and the Occupational Safety and Health Administration (OSHA) controls its exposure in the workplace.

But its use is not controlled in NutraSweet. This sweetener contains seven times more methanol than allowed in any other food product. Products that contain NutraSweet must include a warning that says, "Warning: Phenylketonurics: Contains phenylalanine." This is for people who have a genetic defect that won't allow them to metabolize phenylalanine.

The FDA also publishes a list of the most common side effects associated with the use of this product. Number five is stomach cramps, and number seven is diarrhea. Eliminate this sweetener!

Splenda

Splenda (sucralose) is created by slightly changing sugar's molecular structure through the addition of chlorine.

Manufacturer's Defense. The manufacturer's spin is that it reduces sugar's caloric content using a patented multistep process that selectively replaces three hydrogen-oxygen groups in the sugar molecule with three chlorine atoms. It says that this chlorine molecule is similar to what is found in sodium chloride, or table salt. It also claims that this artificial sweetener isn't absorbed by the body. Seems benign, doesn't it?

The Reality. Chlorine is not chloride. Sodium chloride is table salt; chlorine is found in your swimming pool and in many pesticides, including DDT. The manufacturer's claim that Splenda isn't absorbed by the body is disputed by numerous studies that have shown that 20 to 40 percent of the product is absorbed. Studies have also shown that the sweetener affects weight loss and causes the thymus gland to shrink. While the manufacturer blames the thymus-gland shrinkage on weight loss, studies have shown that simple weight loss does not cause the thymus gland to shrink. Additional studies have linked Splenda to possible liver, kidney, and gastrointestinal problems. No long-term studies have been conducted with Splenda.

Acesulfame K

Acesulfame K is made from a potassium salt. The K stands for potassium.

Manufacturer's Defense. The manufacturer claims that the product is safe.

The Reality. Ever since acesulfame K was first introduced to the market, the Center for Science in the Public Interest has claimed that it has been inadequately tested and is a potential carcinogen (cancer-causing agent). The least used of the artificial sweeteners, it is still too questionable to be considered safe.

But over time, the foods started to cause you problems again and your symptoms slowly returned. Complicating your identification of which food is the culprit are the facts that you reintroduced the foods so long ago and were so initially successful. The solution is to once again implement all your original dietary restrictions. If your symptoms go away, you'll know what caused them, and you'll need to reintroduce your favorite foods much more slowly, if at all.

❖ *You've begun using a different brand of a certain food.* Perhaps the grocery store was out of your regular brand, which never caused you any problems, so you purchased a competing brand. What you didn't notice was that the ingredients were just different enough to cause you problems.

❖ *You've begun taking a new supplement or medication.* Eliminate the supplement and see if your symptoms decrease in severity once more. Discuss with your physician any elimination of new medications.

❖ *You've had to take a course of antibiotics since becoming symptom-free.* If you did, and you forgot to take your probiotics while on the antibiotics and then for one to two months afterward, you've found your problem. See Chapter 4 for the specific probiotics to take.

Conquering IBS can be confusing. There are so many variables, especially when it comes to the food you are eating or anything else you might be ingesting. This process of elimination may not seem to be helpful the first time you read it, but you may be surprised while driving down the street in a day or two. Suddenly something hits you that you didn't think about initially. You are looking for a small detail here, something that doesn't necessarily make sense immediately. Put some thought into this concept, and you may be rewarded with a detail you forgot about or had no idea meant anything.

PSYCHOLOGY AND SYMPTOMS

You may have been suffering from IBS for so long that no matter how much you improve on this program, you'll *expect* your symptoms to return. Especially if your symptoms include loose bowels or diarrhea and you have to take note of every bathroom between your home and your destination whenever you go out, after years of bad experiences due to IBS you've developed a patterned way of thinking. Sort of like Pavlov's dog.

For years, whenever you've needed to leave your home, you've had to make sure that you knew where every single restroom was. Getting in a car is scary, especially to go on a long trip,

The Variables That Cause Symptoms

The main reason that very smart people cannot figure out why they are uncomfortable and having the symptoms they are is because the same symptoms may be caused by different variables in different people. The protocol presented in this book addresses many separate variables, all of which contribute to various gastrointestinal symptoms. You may have two or three variables affecting your system while another person may have seven or eight. The following chart provides a clue to the many variables and the symptoms they cause.

Symptoms	Reduced Good Bacteria	Improper Chemistry	Lack of Digestive Enzymes	Dairy Products	Gas-Causing Foods	Drinking with Meals	Bacteria, Parasites, Yeast	Fructose	Gluten	Food Allergy	Celiac Disease
Gas	✔	✔	✔	✔	✔	✔	✔	✔	✔	✔	✔
Bloating	✔	✔	✔	✔	✔	✔	✔	✔	✔	✔	✔
Indigestion		✔	✔	✔	✔	✔	✔	✔	✔	✔	✔
Heartburn		✔		✔	✔	✔		✔	✔	✔	
Reflux		✔		✔	✔	✔		✔	✔	✔	
Diarrhea	✔	✔		✔			✔	✔	✔	✔	✔
Constipation	✔	✔	✔	✔			✔				
Ulcers		✔					✔				
Pain	✔	✔	✔	✔	✔		✔	✔	✔	✔	✔
Cramping	✔	✔		✔	✔		✔	✔	✔	✔	✔

because you know you have to make pitstops. This patterned way of thinking has become ingrained. But what will happen once you begin to see positive changes on this program?

Many people are grateful and find their quality of life improving dramatically. Some people, however, can't get over their patterned way of thinking no matter how well their bowels work at home, so when they go out, they still have the same old problems. Why? At home, their gastrointestinal systems are perfect, but when they go out for an extended period, they find their old symptoms returning. These folks seem to work themselves up about going out because, after all, it's been years since they could leave the house without symptoms.

The solution to the problem is just to trust. If you have perfect gastrointestinal function at home, you should have it when you go out, and you can. As I mentioned in Chapter 1, stress is not the cause of IBS; it only exacerbates the symptoms. Learning to trust and to calm down before leaving the house will, in time, have you feeling just as comfortable on trips as you are at home.

This may well have been the most important chapter you have read in this book. To have told you what vitamins, minerals, herbs, and other supplements to use, given you the dosages, and left it at that would possibly have been a recipe for failure. IBS is such a complex issue with so many variables to address that without the thought process we have just discussed, your chances for success would be slim. I assure you that somewhere along the way, you'll need to take at least some and possibly all of the advanced steps outlined in this chapter. Read this chapter several times, and refer to it often as you work your way through the supplements, dietary restrictions, and lab tests. The solution to eliminating your symptoms will, in virtually every situation, be found in these steps.

The next chapter will describe why most people with IBS have additional symptoms that are seemingly unrelated to their gastrointestinal systems. We will discuss the wide range of symptoms that most of these people have, the mechanism that causes them, and their relationship to food allergies.

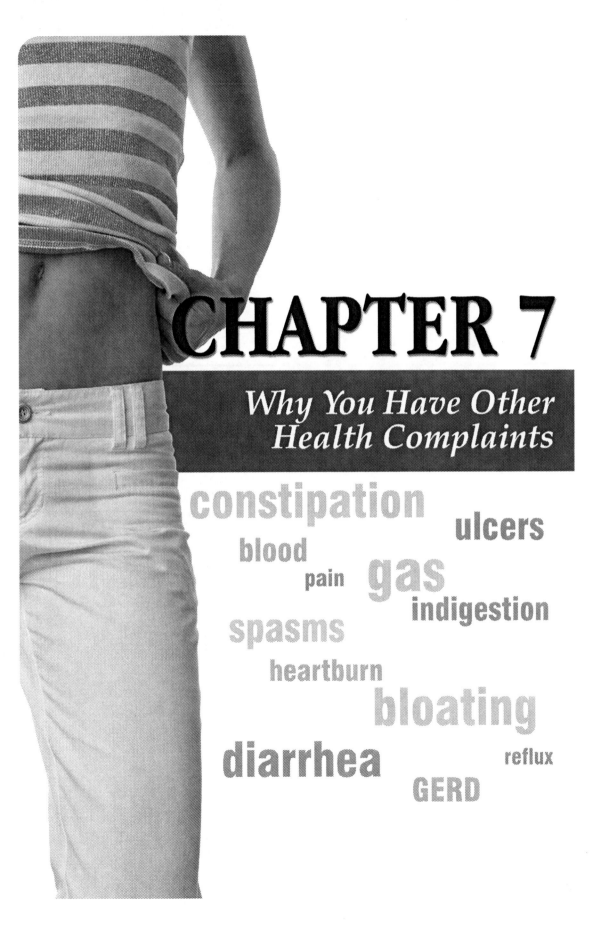

CHAPTER 7

Why You Have Other Health Complaints

constipation

ulcers

blood

pain

gas

indigestion

spasms

heartburn

bloating

diarrhea

reflux

GERD

How do I know you have other health complaints? When new patients come to my office, I always take a complete health history during our initial consultation. More times than not, these new patients report other health complaints. They're in my office for the treatment of IBS, Crohn's Disease or colitis and often feel these other health issues are asides. They feel these other symptoms are not high priorities, especially if they feel they've got them under control with the help of medications. But many of these symptoms are directly related to the function of the gastrointestinal system. In other words, these people wouldn't have those complaints if they didn't have IBS or IBD.

I know your main interest is the elimination of your IBS symptoms, but I think you might find it helpful to understand why you also have other symptoms, if you do. If you don't have any additional health complaints,

Case History: Miranda

Miranda presented in my office complaining of headaches, asthma, and chronic sinus infections. She was 57 years old, 5 feet 4 inches tall, and weighed 135 pounds. She had always considered herself a relatively healthy person. The headaches were becoming more frequent, and she was using more of her asthma medication than she used to. She was about 20 pounds heavier than she was 20 years ago.

After discussing her history and current symptoms, Miranda was quite surprised and a bit embarrassed when I began asking her questions about her bowel habits. I explained that the information was more important than she realized, and she admitted she alternated between weeks of diarrhea and weeks of what she considered normal bowels. She self-medicated with Imodium when she went through a period of diarrhea.

Miranda was very eager to start my protocol, which made returning her bowels to normal the cornerstone of a treatment plan for the other symptoms she had come to me about. She said my explanation made quite a bit of sense to her and wondered

(continued on page 94)

(continued from page 93)

why any of her other doctors had not take that approach. She was extremely interested in learning as much as she could about leaky gut syndrome and the role that histamine played in causing her non-gastrointestinal symptoms.

I advised her to begin my inflammatory bowel disease protocol (see Chapter Nine), using the supplements, following the dietary eliminations, and testing for food allergies. Miranda's bowels became better formed in a relatively short time, and her sinus congestion cleared within weeks. Her headaches resolving in slightly more than one week made her the happiest. The asthma was a little more difficult to solve, but we continued to meet every so often and each time she reported she was using less and less of her sinus medications and inhalers. In fact, she couldn't even remember the last time she had used her rescue inhaler. A bonus was increased energy and weight loss.

you'll learn another reason it's important to eliminate IBS and stop the process from continuing to a point where you may experience additional symptoms in the future.

When your gastrointestinal system becomes unhealthy, a cascade of events is set into motion. The loss of the beneficial bacteria population leads to a change in chemistry, which leads to the development of unhealthy tissue, which in turn leads to low-level inflammation. In this chapter, we'll discuss where this low-level inflammation leads.

THE ROLE OF HISTAMINE

If we could actually get into your small intestine and look closely at the tissue, we would see that it looks unhealthy and has low-level inflammation. When tissue becomes inflamed, it also expands. The same way that a bad sunburn causes the skin on the outside of the body to swell and the pores to enlarge, inflammation of the tissue on the inside of the gastrointestinal system, particularly in the small intestine, also causes swelling and "holes." During a colonoscopy, a doctor can take a sample of this tissue—that is, slice off a small piece of tissue from the lining of the small intestine—which can then be placed under a microscope for the purpose of identifying any abnormalities, including swelling, inflammation, and holes between the cells. Conventional medicine calls this condition malabsorption syndrome. In alternative or holistic medicine, it's called leaky gut syndrome. No, nothing is leaking out of you, but foods and bacterial enzymes may be leaking into your bloodstream.

You already know that you aren't digesting your food properly. The most common symptoms associated with undigested food are gas, bloating, indigestion, heartburn, nausea, pain, and cramping. If you are experiencing any of these symptoms, you can safely assume that you aren't digesting your food properly and that undigested foods are being absorbed, in abnormal amounts, through the lining of your small intestine. Even if you aren't experiencing any of the symptoms commonly associated with not digesting your food properly (by "properly," I mean completely and within a specific amount of time), you may still be experiencing problems at a cellular level.

Through normal digestion, food is broken down into its various components. In a normal gastrointestinal system, these individual molecules are absorbed from cell to cell to cell till they reach the bloodstream.

In an unhealthy gastrointestinal system, foods that haven't yet been fully broken down will pass through the holes in the intestinal wall (rather than moving from cell to cell) into the capillary bed of the circulatory system (the bloodstream). No, we're not talking about chunks of chicken or pieces of cheese. We're talking microscopically. The circulatory system is in charge of transporting the nutritional components of the foods you eat throughout your body, not pieces of undigested food.

In the bloodstream, the body doesn't expect to encounter undigested food. It looks for the basic components of food—the vitamins, minerals, fatty acids, and such—in the form of separate molecules, not as molecules that have not been separated from each other. While it's able to recognize separate molecules, it doesn't have the ability to recognize groups of molecules. Therefore, it places a call to the immune system to come over, inspect the newcomers, and take appropriate action. The most important part of this story—and the part that most affects you—is the next step. When the immune system is called into action, the first thing it does is create an antibody to the group of molecules it finds. Then, as it works to identify what it has found, it generates the release of a number of chemicals, including one called *histamine*.

SYMPTOMS CAUSED BY HISTAMINE

Did you notice how I italicized the word *histamine*? Think I'm trying to tell you something? It's that important.

Most people know what an antihistamine is. You've probably used one yourself. An antihistamine relieves allergy symptoms, such as runny nose, stuffiness, and red eyes. That means that *histamine* must cause those symptoms. Guess what else *histamine* causes in the body? Look at the list in the chapter that names all the symptoms that have been associated with *histamine* and food allergies. That list is long! The most common symptoms it includes are headaches, pain and inflammation, skin rashes, psoriasis, eczema, hives, irregular heartbeat, asthma, and anaphylactic shock (hampered breathing possibly leading to death). Not all of these symptoms occur in everyone, but depending on a person's biochemical individuality, some or all may appear.

In addition to causing symptoms, histamine also acts as a sort of assistant in chronic infections such as sinusitis, bronchitis, yeast infection, urinary tract infection, nail or toe fungus, athlete's foot, and jock itch. The more your immune system has to work overtime to combat culinary invaders, the less time and energy it has to combat your body's other infections. This may be why you have certain infections over and over again. It may also explain the existence of autoimmune diseases, because an overactive immune system may be more easily confused between what is normal tissue and what is not.

FOOD ALLERGIES

Now you know the mechanism inside the gastrointestinal system that allows the creation of a food allergy. Unfortunately, your favorite foods in particular are the ones that are crossing over into your bloodstream and creating this chain of events. If we have tissue that allows food particles, regardless of size, to move from the inside of your small intestine into the bloodstream, it makes perfect sense that the foods you eat the most have the greatest opportunity to create an immune reaction. Said another way, you cannot be allergic to foods you don't eat. Please see Food Allergy Testing in the Laboratory Tests section of the Resource List at the back of this book.

If you're like most people, when you go shopping you go to the same stores each time and always buy the same brands. People like their familiar choices. These foods—your favorites—are the ones that are passing through your leaky gut and causing your food allergies. Part of becoming well is to make different food choices while you rebalance your gastrointestinal system using the protocol described in this book.

It's amazing how many other conditions my office patients report having in addition to IBS. In this chapter, we examined the mechanism responsible for the creation of these other symp-

Common Symptoms of Histamine Release

Conventional medicine has quite a bit of knowledge about histamine. How it's created and its systemic effects are well documented in medical textbooks. The connection between foods, histamine, and the many health conditions linked to it are not as well understood by the average physician. You might recognize the skin conditions listed below because you have taken antihistamine medications such as Benedryl for them. Note the additional health conditions also linked to histamine.

Autoimmune Symptoms
Ankylosing Spondylitis
Multiple sclerosis
Rheumatoid arthritis
Systemic lupus erythematosus

Dermatologic Symptoms
Acne
Canker sores
Dermatitis
Eczema
Hives
Itching
Rash

Gastrointestinal Symptoms
Abdominal pain and colic
Celiac disease
Crohn's disease
Constipation
Diarrhea
Duodenal ulcer
Functional intestinal obstruction
Gas
Gastritis
Infantile colic
Intestinal hemorrhage
Irritable bowel syndrome
Loss of appetite
Malabsorption
Ulcerative colitis
Vomiting
Weight gain

General Symptoms
Anemia
Fainting
Hypoglycemia
Sinusitis

Genitourinary Symptoms
Bedwetting
Chronic bladder infections
Nephrosis (kidney disease)

Immune System Symptoms
Chronic or recurrent yeast infections
Chronic or recurrent urinary tract infections
Chronic or recurrent ear infections
Chronic or recurrent sinus infections
Chronic or recurrent bronchitis

Musculoskeletal Symptoms
Bursitis
Joint pain
Low back pain

Neurological Symptoms
Anaphylactic shock
Asthma
Chronic rhinitis
Coughing and wheezing
Fatigue
Headache
Recurrent bronchitis
Recurrent croup
Recurrent otitis media

toms, so now you not only know why you have them, but that you'll probably see them improve or even disappear once you eliminate your IBS symptoms.

If you also have children with IBS, the next chapter will guide you in helping them. Children are much easier to treat than adults and respond to this program much more quickly.

CHAPTER 8

IBS in Children and Teens

constipation

ulcers

blood

pain

gas

indigestion

spasms

heartburn

bloating

diarrhea

reflux

GERD

First, the great news all parents want to hear is that children and teens respond very quickly to the program described in this book. In fact, the younger they are, the quicker they respond. Second, and even better, they might not need all the products I suggest for adults, nor will they need to be on the program as long.

It seems that the inherent resiliency and strength of youth coupled with the rapid rate of growth means that the changes that need to occur for health to return happen much faster than in adults. I've seen it time and again in my office. Worried parents want a solution to their child's misery and discomfort. We make the necessary dietary changes and begin the product protocol, and the child reports an end to the problems seemingly overnight. So, how do we do that for your child? In this chapter, we'll discuss how to take the program for adults and tweak it for children and teens.

THE BIG FOUR DON'T-YOU-*DARE*-BREAK-'EM DIETARY RULES

Like adults, children and teens with IBS report having the more common symptoms of gas, bloating, indigestion, heartburn, diarrhea, constipation, and even vomiting. The younger the children, the more they also seem to suffer from stomachaches. The reason they have these symptoms and what can be done about them are the same as for adults.

As already discussed, antibiotics are the primary cause of IBS, though possibly not the only cause. They alter the bacterial balance of the gastrointestinal system, leading to a change in chemistry, which leads to symptoms and, more than likely, food intolerances or allergies to favorite foods.

Like adults, children should begin this program by following the dietary eliminations described in Chapter 5. Again, the most important elimination is dairy. I know it'll be tough. Your child will complain, and all you'll want to do is give in to him or her. However, please be tough.

Case History: Katie

Children want to eat their favorite foods. Isn't that a parental pleasure—to give your children not only healthy foods, but ones that make them happy? What if they love dairy products and gluten-containing foods and foods they tested allergic to? Parents have a difficult time with this.

Katie was 12 years old and had been diagnosed with Crohn's disease. She had been hospitalized a number of times because of the diarrhea, bleeding, and dehydration she was experiencing. Her mother contacted me as a last resort.

I explained to Katie's mother that children respond much quicker than adults and with the use of less supplements if my protocol is followed to the letter. Katie's mother agreed to follow my advice and to also have Katie tested for allergies. During our second meeting, to go over the results of the allergy test, Katie's mother told me they were not totally following the no-dairy and no-gluten rules. Katie had been complaining, saying she had nothing to eat, and threw a little temper tantrum once in a while. Mom wanted to keep the peace and struggled with not giving Katie the foods she wanted. I knew we had a hurdle to get over or the allergy test results would also be an obstacle.

I explained the test results and attempted to motivate Mom to do better with Katie's diet. Not only should Katie avoid dairy and gluten, but there were also a number of foods she was allergic to, and a couple of them she ate regularly.

(continued on page 104)

Dairy is the main villain for everyone with gastrointestinal complaints, but especially for children. And especially for children with stomachaches.

If following the Big Four Don't-You-*Dare*-Break-'Em Dietary Rules doesn't completely eliminate your child's complaints, remember that you may very well have to work your way through the fructose and gluten eliminations described in Chapter 6.

THE SUPPLEMENTS

The product protocol for children and teens is a bit different than that for adults. From among the supplements discussed in Chapter 4, you should definitely use the essential supplements to reestablish bacterial balance and the essential supplements to feed the tissue and restore chemistry. You will need to reestablish the population of beneficial bacteria (probiotics), and you will also need to feed the tissue in the gastrointestinal system to restore its health, just like in adults. Whether or not to use the essential supplements to improve digestion and restore pH or any of the supplements for special circumstances will be a judgment call you'll need to make. (See "The Optional Supplements," below.)

To reestablish the beneficial bacteria population in children and teens, use the same *Lactobacillus* and *Bifidobacterium* products recommended for adults. However, use them as follows:

- ❖ For children under 5 years old, use one half of the adult dosage of each product once a day for two to three weeks.

- ❖ For children aged 5 to 10 years, use the full adult dosage of each product once a day for one month.

- ❖ For children over 10 years old, use the full adult dosage of each product twice a day for one month.

If you child can't swallow pills, buy a form of product that can be dissolved in water or put into cold food. Remember to give your child the supplements on an empty stomach and to buy probiotics that need to be refrigerated.

To feed the tissue and restore the chemistry of the gastrointestinal system in children and teens, use the same rice protein powder, glutamine, other amino acids, inulin, and FOS products discussed in Chapter 4. However, use them as follows:

- ❖ For children under 5 years old, use one fourth of the adult dosage of each product twice a day for two to three weeks.

- ❖ For children aged 5 to 10 years, use one half of the adult dosage of each product twice a day for one month.

- ❖ For children over 10 years old, use the full adult dosage of each product twice a day for one to two months.

None of the above time frames is set in stone. Your child may need to take the supplements a bit longer than recommended. It will depend on your child's age and symptoms. The older the child, the longer it may take to completely heal and repair the gastrointestinal system.

Don't be afraid of overdosing your child. These supplements in these amounts are safe and don't have side effects. Keep in mind, however, that if gas or bloating increases, you may need to have a stool test done. For information about stool testing, see Chapters 6 and the Laboratory Tests section in the Resource List at the back of the book.

THE OPTIONAL SUPPLEMENTS

Under most circumstances, the other products used by adults (the essential supplements to improve digestion and restore pH and the supplements for special circumstances) are not need-

(continued from page 102)

I let it go for another couple of weeks, until Katie's next appointment. When I saw them next, Katie and her mom were disappointed, as Katie had been hospitalized since I had last seen her. Now was the time to more strongly suggest that Mom was in charge and that it was her responsibility to follow my advice. I told her that if she didn't, we were just chasing our tails. I also had a heart-to-heart--as best I could--with Katie about the importance of letting Mom tell her what she could and could not eat. It was "just for now," I said. She would get back her favorite foods in a short while.

Katie and her mother both understood the serious nature of what we were facing. They followed the protocol to the letter, and Katie's progress became astonishing. Her bowels became normal in a few weeks, and she went off all her anti-inflammatory prescription medications in a few months. Katie didn't like it, but she was a trooper and did what she needed to do.

I can't tell you how many times I have had parents who, wanting to give their children only the best and what made them happy, had a very difficult time restricting certain food villains. It always pains them greatly to see the children complain and, worse yet, cry. But they are the parents and it is their responsibility to provide the best food for their children. Sometimes the best thing a parent can do is refuse to allow their child to eat the foods they love the most.

ed by children. For teens under 16 years old, you'll need to make a judgment call. See if your child finds relief without them. If, after a few weeks, your child has been following all the dietary restrictions and taking all the recommended supplements, you've worked your way through the step-by-step thought process as adjusted for children, and your child is still complaining of gas, bloating, heartburn, or reflux, add these other products into the mix. For teens 16 years old and over, these products might very well be necessary, just to make sure you cover all your bases. Use the adult dosages for these older teens.

THE LABORATORY TESTS

With younger office patients, I save the lab tests for last. That doesn't mean your child won't need them. It just means that I recommend waiting before you spend the time and money because the majority of my younger patients see a complete elimination of their symptoms just by following the protocol described above. If your child doesn't see results, or doesn't see good enough results, you can always have the lab work done later.

Take heart, and have hope. I know how heart-wrenching it is to see your child sick. However, the simple protocol described in this chapter will work wonders. All it involves is giving your child supplements to reestablish a normal bacterial balance and restore proper chemistry, combined with following some temporary dietary restrictions. It's less complex than what adults need to do, and it usually works in much less time.

In the next chapter, we'll discuss how to treat Crohn's Disease and any type of colitis for both adults and children.

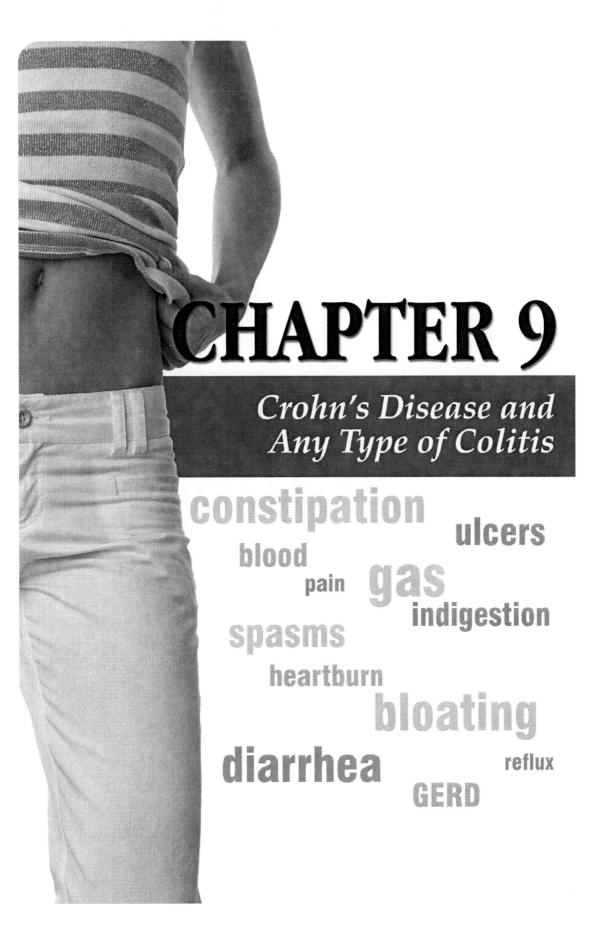

CHAPTER 9

Crohn's Disease and Any Type of Colitis

constipation

ulcers

blood

pain

gas

indigestion

spasms

heartburn

bloating

diarrhea

reflux

GERD

I am asked all the time, "How do you know if I have Crohn's disease or one of the types of colitis?" It's simple. If you have not been formally diagnosed with Crohn's disease or a type of colitis, then the information in this chapter is not for you. If you have not heard your physician tell you that you have one of the conditions described in this chapter, please consider yourself an irritable bowel syndrome patient and follow the advice in this book about IBS.

Is it possible that Crohn's disease and any form of colitis, also known as inflammatory bowel diseases (IBD), are just advanced cases of irritable bowel syndrome? Do all cases of Crohn's disease and any form of colitis begin with IBS? If you have Crohn's disease or colitis, did you ignore the symptoms that preceded their full-fledged development and allow them to advance to the more serious condition? Have you been misdiagnosed?

Case History: Richard

Richard was 35 years old, 6 feet 4 inches tall, and 210 pounds—well, at least he used to be. When he came to my office with ulcerative colitis, he weighed 175 pounds. He was experiencing diarrhea with blood and mucus ten or more times each day. He didn't know what to eat. Everything he ate hurt him and so he avoided food. He was scared and had nowhere left to turn.

Richard was a patient in my office at a time when I did not call for a food allergy test for all my inflammatory bowel disease patients. And I struggled to get them well. Richard is responsible for the change in protocol that now allows me to claim such a significant success record.

Struggle we did, and more than two months into the protocol, we decided to test Richard for food allergies. The results came back, and surprisingly, we discovered he was not allergic to many foods. The food he was most allergic to was olives. When I went through the results and informed him of that, he started to laugh and said, "My wife is Italian and puts olive oil on everything".

(continued on page 110)

(continued from page 109)

Within two weeks of giving up olive oil and the few other foods to which he was found to be allergic, his stools were well-formed and he moved his bowels just a couple of times each day, with no blood or mucus. In two months, he gained back 20 pounds.

From that moment on, I began to strongly advise all my Crohn's disease and colitis patients to have the test for food allergies at the beginning of my protocol. As a result, my success record has skyrocketed. Please note that olives are considered a healthy food unless you are allergic to them. After a short period of avoiding them, you can add them back to your diet again. Also, be advised that we all have different allergies and this example is not meant to suggest that you should give up olives.

I believe that Crohn's disease and any type of colitis both begin with symptoms that are very similar, if not identical, to those of IBS. More than likely, the early symptoms are allowed to progress either because they're ignored or because they're able to advance thanks to the use of ineffective treatment protocols. I don't have any proof of this; it simply makes sense. You can consider Crohn's Disease and any type of colitis just to be an advanced deterioration of the balance and function of your gastrointestinal system. You need not consider it a disease, it's a condition that can go away.

Adding weight to my argument is that in my practice, I have almost the same success rate with Crohn's disease and all types of colitis that I do with IBS. Let me repeat that: *I have almost the same success rate with Crohn's disease and all types of colitis that I do with IBS*. Like IBS patients, people with either of these conditions need to reestablish their proper bacterial levels, restore their proper chemistry, and identify and eliminate from their diet the foods that are contributing to the inflammatory process going on in their gastrointestinal system. However, there are differences between my IBS protocol and my treatment protocol for Crohn's disease and colitis, and we'll discuss them in this chapter.

WHAT ARE CROHN'S DISEASE AND COLITIS?

First, let's talk about Crohn's disease and the many forms of colitis. You may have a diagnosis of one of these conditions, so an understanding of exactly what they are may be helpful. My perspective is that neither Crohn's nor any type of colitis is a disease. They are "conditions" of the gastrointestinal system in which the ultimate health and balance of the tissue has changed for the worse. It is a severe deterioration of the balance of your gastrointestinal system. This then suggests, and my experience proves correct, that the lack of health and the imbalance can be reversed.

There are differences between Crohn's and colitis, but the similarities between the conditions are what is important to remember. They both have as clinical findings inflamed tissue and immune-system involvement contributing to that inflammation. Even with their differences, the treatment presented in this book works for both Crohn's disease and all the types of colitis.

Crohn's Disease

Crohn's disease can affect any area of the gastrointestinal tract, but it most commonly affects the lower part of the small intestine, called the ileum. The swelling extends deep into the lining of the tissue of the gastrointestinal system, causing pain and other uncomfortable symptoms. The condition is also called ileitis and enteritis. Crohn's Disease is also a condition that involves the immune system.

In Crohn's disease, normal healthy bowel can be found between sections of diseased bowel. The disease affects men and women equally and seems to run in some families. About 20 percent of people with Crohn's disease have a blood relative, most often a brother or sister and sometimes a parent or child, with some form of inflammatory bowel disease. Crohn's disease can occur in people of all age groups, but it is more often diagnosed in people between the ages of twenty and thirty and especially of Jewish heritage.

Ulcerative Colitis

Ulcerative colitis is a condition that causes inflammation and sores, called ulcers, in the top layer of the lining of the rectum and colon. Ulcers form where inflammation has killed the cells that usually line the colon. They then bleed and produce pus. Ulcerative colitis is also a condition that involves the immune system.

When the inflammation occurs in the rectum and lower part of the colon, it is called ulcerative proctitis. If the entire colon is affected, it is called pancolitis. If only the left side of the colon is affected, it is called limited or distal colitis.

Ulcerative colitis can occur in people of any age, but it usually starts between the ages of fifteen and thirty, and less frequently between fifty and seventy years of age. It affects men and women equally and appears to run in families, with reports of up to 20 percent of people with ulcerative colitis having a family member or relative with ulcerative colitis or Crohn's disease. A higher incidence of ulcerative colitis is seen in Caucasians and people of Jewish descent.

Collagenous, Lymphocytic, and Microscopic Colitis

Collagenous and lymphocytic colitis are also called microscopic colitis. In microscopic colitis, there is no sign of inflammation on the surface of the colon when viewed during a colonoscopy, a test that lets a doctor look inside the large intestine. Because the inflammation isn't visible, a biopsy is necessary to make a diagnosis. In this biopsy, a small piece of tissue from the lining of the intestine is removed during a colonoscopy.

The immune system is also involved in microscopic colitis. The characteristic feature of lymphocytic colitis is the presence of an abundance of white blood cells, suggesting an infection. Collagenous colitis shares this feature but additionally shows a distinctive thickening of the tissue lining the colon.

Pseudomembranous Colitis

Pseudomembranous colitis is an acute inflammatory condition of the colon that in mild cases may appear as minimal inflammation or swelling of the lining of the colon. In more severe cases, the lining often is covered with raised bumps that look yellowish.

Ischemic Colitis

Ischemic colitis is an unusual type of colitis, more rare than the other types, and characterized by a lack of blood flow to the tissue in parts of the colon. Occurring more at an older age, this type of colitis has a cause more related to heart disease or atherosclerosis (hardening of the arteries). Positive response to the protocol in this book would not be as dramatic or frequent as for the other types of colitis or Crohn's disease.

DIFFERENCES BETWEEN THE PROTOCOLS

My protocol for treating IBS differs in two primary ways from my protocol for treating Crohn's disease and any of the types of colitis. Crohn's disease and colitis are inflammatory conditions, which IBS isn't. To treat the inflammation, we will add some all-natural anti-inflammatory herbs and other compounds to the mix of essential supplements. In addition, Crohn's disease and colitis have an immune-system component that IBS doesn't. Therefore, I recommend eliminating all gluten-containing foods from your diet and having a food allergy test at the beginning of the program instead of toward the end, as I suggest for people with IBS (if they need it at all). At this point, it's important to understand the steps you need to take. The steps to help you with inflammatory bowel disease (IBD) are similar to those I have already outlined for IBS. Begin all of the following steps immediately.

Begin The Essential Supplements

The protocol for IBD uses the same supplements as the IBS protocol, described in Chapter 4. Please review that chapter for this information. Use the supplements for a minimum of three months to reestablish beneficial bacteria, feed the tissue, restore chemistry, improve digestion, and restore pH. After three months, you probably won't need the supplements to improve digestion and restore pH any longer, but you can make the call on that. However, continue to use the other supplements until you have completely gone off your medications and for one to two months after. (Please see "Stopping Your Medications" at the end of this chapter.)

Add Anti-Inflammatory Supplements

Irritable bowel syndrome, like Crohn's disease and colitis, usually involves some level of inflammation somewhere in the gastrointestinal tract. In Crohn's disease and colitis, however, the inflammation is more advanced. Therefore, to successfully treat Crohn's disease and colitis, we need to eliminate the inflammation in addition to halting the immune system's involvement.

The best way to treat the inflammation of Crohn's disease and colitis is with all-natural anti-inflammatory supplements, which unlike medications won't add any of their own side effects to the mix. Two herbs that I always recommend to my office patients are ginger and turmeric. Both ginger and turmeric have been used for centuries because of their anti-inflammatory properties, and they have also been found to be antibacterial and to have antioxidant properties. Their anti-inflammatory properties function by inhibiting the chemistry associated with the cyclooxygenase (COX) enzymes. These are the same enzymes inhibited by medications such as Celebrex.

Other good anti-inflammatory compounds to try are citrulline, D-limonene, rosemary leaf extract, hesperidin, rutin, and quercetin. These compounds act synergistically to help with the healing process. Take them as follows:

❖ 100 milligrams of ginger root extract *(Zingiber officinale)*, standardized to 5-percent (5 milligrams) of the total pungent compounds

❖ 210 milligrams of turmeric rhizome extract *(Curcuma longa)*, standardized to 95-percent (200 milligrams) of the total pungent compounds

❖ 100 milligrams each of citrulline, D-limonene, and rosemary leaf extract

❖ 200 milligrams each of hesperidin, rutin, and quercetin

Take each of these additional supplements twice a day.

Follow the Big Four Dietary Rules

You should begin using the essential supplements and anti-inflammatory supplements and make changes to your diet all at the same time. Please review Chapter 5 for the rules regarding the elimination of dairy products, beans and legumes, and fruit; drinking liquids during meals or up to one hour afterwards; and discontinuing the use of vitamin supplements.

Please note that the rules about eliminating beans and legumes and no liquids or fruits to be eaten during a meal or for one hour after are to improve your digestion and help you eliminate gas and bloating. They are NOT essential to conquering Crohn's Disease and colitis. Most of my patients come to me with complaints of gas and bloating, so these two rules simply identify and eliminate a variable possibly responsible for these symptoms. If you don't have complaints of gas and bloating or are vegetarian, you can adjust this rule to your needs.

Eliminate Gluten

One additional food group that is important for people with Crohn's disease and colitis to eliminate from the get-go is gluten-containing foods. After many years and thousands of patients, I have found that in almost all cases, gluten is a villain that must be avoided because of its effects on the gastrointestinal system.

Gluten is contained in foods such as wheat, oats, barley, and rye. This is also a 100-percent elimination, as there will be no room for allowing any in your diet. If a food from a package, bottle, can, box, or frozen convenience food has an ingredient list, read it before you begin eating.

Wheat is made into flour and may be called white flour, whole wheat flour, bleached flour, or unbleached flour on an ingredient list. Breads, cookies, cakes, crackers, bagels, and pasta are some foods that contain wheat. You will also find wheat added to other convenience or frozen foods. If the food is breaded, it's breaded with wheat. Gluten is also found on dried fruits, as they are coated with flour to prevent sticking. Certain sauces and condiments may contain modified food starch, another gluten product.

Oatmeal contains oats, as does granola. Many breakfast bars and protein bars also contain oats.

Barley is found as a grain added to vegetable and other soups, and is also made into regular or white vinegar. As a substitute for white vinegar, use apple cider vinegar, balsamic vinegar or rice vinegar. If you find the word "malt" in an ingredient list, avoid the product, as malt also comes from barley.

Staying away from rye is very easy, as you will almost always find it only in rye bread, which is made from wheat flour with rye flour added.

Have a Food Allergy Test

IBS, Crohn's disease and any type of colitis are all disorders of the gastrointestinal system. One of the two things that make Crohn's disease and colitis different from IBS is the involvement of the immune system. This involvement is important to understand because some of the most common foods you eat may contribute to the inflammatory process.

Unhealthy gastrointestinal systems swell and leave "holes" between the cells. Food not yet fully digested "falls" through the holes in the intestinal wall rather than continuing through the intestines and becoming fully digested—that is, broken down

Stool Testing and the Presence of Abnormal Organisms

In the IBS sections of this book, I make references to the use of stool testing, which is discussed at length in the Laboratory Tests section in the Resource List at the back of this book. People with Crohn's disease or colitis seem to rarely need stool testing. I have no idea why.

It seems to be a much larger problem with IBS, with about a third of the people with this disorder needing this helpful evaluation. The only reason I can come up with—and I have no scientific backing to base this on—is that the environment within the gastrointestinal system of people with IBD is so unhealthy that even these villainous organisms don't wish to live there. Or, they simply can't.

Crohn's Disease and Any Type of Colitis in Children and Teens

Worried parents contact my office everyday to ask one simple question: "Will your protocol help my child, and is it safe?" The answer is absolutely yes. And the really wonderful news is that kids respond so much more quickly to this protocol than adults and with lower amounts of supplements.

I believe the reason for the amazing success of this protocol in younger people is their incredible rate of growth. Childrens' and teenagers' metabolisms are so fast that anything we do to improve their diet and the environment inside their gastrointestinal system shows positive effects in very short order. This makes restoration of beneficial bacteria levels and improvements in inflamed tissue much easier.

The essential supplement protocol for children with Crohn's disease and any type of colitis is the same as it is for adults, except that young people have no need for the supplements used to improve digestion and restore pH. Their gastrointestinal systems are probably producing more than adequate amounts of digestive enzymes. They will need the food allergy test.

Add to the essential supplements the anti-inflammatory supplements mentioned earlier in this chapter. Use one third of the dose for children under five, one half of the dose for children between six and ten, and the full dose for children over ten. These all-natural products have no side effects.

Use these supplements until you see your child's symptoms go away, then continue using them while you wean the child off his or her medications, along with your physician's help, using one of the methods described earlier in this chapter. Once the child is off the medications, use the recommended supplements for an additional month.

into its components of vitamins, minerals, fatty acids, amino acids, and so on. Once through the holes, it enters the bloodstream.

The body doesn't expect or recognize the partially digested pieces of food in the bloodstream, and alerts the immune system to spring into action and create antibodies and chemical substances that have gastrointestinal consequences. In other words, they contribute to the inflammation of the lining of the tissue in the gastrointestinal tract.

Because of the more prominent role that food allergy plays in Crohn's disease and any type of colitis, I recommend having a food allergy test done at the beginning of the program to identify the foods that have created antibodies and chemistry in your bloodstream and are contributing to the inflammatory process. Once you know what these foods are, you should avoid them for at least six months and possibly longer. For a discussion of food allergy testing and how to interpret the test results, see the Laboratory Tests section in the Resource List at the back of this book.

Eliminate Fructose

As with IBS patients, we are finding more and more that a subset of IBD patients are having trouble with foods that contain fructose. I realize that I have already asked you to give up dairy and gluten containing foods, as well as the foods to which you are sensitive according to food allergy testing, but if after trying my protocol for a month or two you find you still have uncomfortable symptoms and have progressed only so far, eliminate fructose from your diet, especially if you eat a lot of foods containing fructose.

Another clue may be that you constantly complain that some of the foods listed in the next paragraph seem to cause you discomfort. Some patients complain that fruits bother them, while others know full well that each time they eat anything sweet, they have gastrointestinal symptoms. That's your body talking to you and clueing you in that you need to make a change. The only way to find out is to stop eating the suspect food.

Fructose is contained in fruit, anything sweet (such as table sugar, honey, molasses, and maple syrup), corn, high fructose corn syrup, beets, carrots, peas, onions, tomatoes, eggplant, sweet potatoes, turnips and winter squash (acorn, buttercup, calabaza, delicata, Hubbard, spaghetti, sweet dumpling, and turban). You should know if this is effective within two to three weeks, sometimes less.

Stop complaining! You still have beef, chicken, fish, pork, eggs, any vegetable not on the above list (about thirty), all types of rice, white and red potatoes, lettuce, spinach, and nuts. That's plenty; anybody can live on that diet.

How to Stop Taking Prescription Medications

"Should I go off my prednisone, mesalamine (Pentasa, Asacol, Rowasa), colazal, 6-mercapturine, azathioprine (Imuran), or methotrexate?" This is a common question in my office, since most patients want to eliminate as many prescription medications as possible and as soon as possible, because of their side effects and because they often don't do a very good job of providing symptom relief. You need to exercise extreme caution here. *Never discontinue taking any prescription medication without first consulting your doctor.*

WHY DOESN'T MY DOCTOR KNOW THIS?

Conquering Irritable Bowel Syndrome, Inflammatory Bowel Disease, Crohn's Disease, and Colitis

Among my office patients, a good number do choose to discontinue taking their prescription medications. However, they do it with medical guidance, and they do it in a very slow, methodical, and conservative way. It makes no difference whether the process takes six weeks or six months. What matters is that it's done safely. So, if *you and your doctor* decide to try to get you off your medications, here's the method I have seen other patients do successfully with their doctor's help.

While still taking your medications, begin the IBS program described in this book with the adjustments for Crohn's disease and colitis described in this chapter. Before you even consider attempting to wean yourself from your medications, you will need to see progress in the form of visible positive changes for two months at a minimum.

If you're lucky, you will notice changes within a few days to a few weeks. These may be in the form of fewer bowel movements each day, reduced bowel urgency, more solid, consistent stool formation, or a lessening of blood or mucus in the stool. If you're unlucky, you may need a while longer to see any improvements or to identify all the foods that may be contributing to your symptoms.

Once you're satisfied that you've been experiencing progress for at least a couple of months, you'll need to decide how to wean yourself off your medications. The method that seems to be preferred by my office patients who take just one medication is to reduce the daily dosage of the medication by about 20 to 25 percent. For example, if you're taking six 400-milligram tablets of Asacol (the common dosage in the early stage of treatment for Crohn's disease or colitis) or four 400-milligram tablets (a common maintenance dosage) per day, decrease your daily dosage by one tablet. Take five or three tablets, respectively, per day for about two to three weeks, then assess your symptoms. If your symptoms have not worsened, reduce your daily dosage by one more tablet, and assess your symptoms again in another two to three weeks. Continue to decrease your daily dosage this way until you're down to zero tablets.

The method that my office patients who take two or more medications seem to prefer involves decreasing the dosage of each medication in turn. For example, if you're taking two medications, decrease the dosage of one as described above until you're taking 50 percent of the original dosage, then decrease the second medication the same way. Repeat the procedure, alternating between the two medications, until you're no longer taking either one.

What's the worst thing that can happen to you if you try to wean yourself off your medications in a slow, methodical, conservative manner and with a doctor's guidance? If at some point you notice that your symptoms are on the upswing again, you can either stop decreasing your dosages or you can increase them again to the previous level. You may have decreased your dosages too quickly for your specific condition. Stay at those previous levels for a month or so, to give the supplements and dietary restrictions more time to make positive changes, then try to move forward again.

Crohn's disease and colitis are cousins of IBS, as far as I'm concerned. They have an immune component that IBS doesn't, plus they're inflammatory conditions, but this doesn't create a problem for my protocol. It just means we need to tweak it a little bit.

In the next chapter, we will discuss a self-massage technique that brings relief from a very common complaint in people with IBS—hiatal hernia.

CHAPTER 10

Hiatal Hernia

constipation

ulcers

blood

pain

gas

indigestion

spasms

heartburn

bloating

diarrhea

reflux

GERD

*I*n addition to the typical symptoms, many people with IBS report that they've also been diagnosed with a hiatal hernia. In this chapter, we'll explain exactly what a hiatal hernia is and describe a self-massage technique that has brought a number of people welcome relief.

WHAT IS A HIATAL HERNIA?

First, a lesson in anatomy. The esophagus is a tubelike organ that connects the mouth to the stomach. Its sole purpose is to act as a conduit for food. It begins at the throat, travels through a muscle called the diaphragm located at the top of the abdomen, and ends at the stomach. A valve at its bottom called the esophageal sphincter opens to allow food to pass through to the stomach, then shuts to prevent the food and stomach acid from spilling from the stomach back into the esophagus.

A hiatal hernia is a condition in which the top of the stomach has slid through the opening of the diaphragm and become stuck. This causes the bottom part of the esophagus to become deformed, which prevents the esophageal sphincter from closing properly and protecting the esophagus from stomach acid. The end result is a host of symptoms including heartburn, pain, and esophageal spasms, as well as the potential for inflammation, Barrett's esophagitis, and esophageal ulcers.

What causes this structural defect to occur? No one knows for sure. The popular theories include the opening of the diaphragm being abnormally large, the esophagus having become shortened due to inflammation and scarring from reflux or GERD, and the esophagus being too loosely attached to the diaphragm. My belief is that hiatal hernia occurs only in people with unhealthy gastrointestinal systems. I believe the cause is, once again, a loss of bacterial balance and proper chemistry which leads to all the imbalances and symptoms we have talked about in this book. If you have a hiatal hernia, my program will help reestablish your bacterial balance and restore your chemistry. But the use of this self massage technique will accelerate the process.

The same as for most chronic health problems, conventional medical doctors have no solution for this painful condition. But there is something you can try. Back in the 1970s, an old chiropractor taught me a self-massage technique that helped my own hiatal hernia resolve. I was a young man when suddenly I began experiencing excruciating pain in my stomach area virtually every day and seemingly all day long. The pain was so severe at times that it would drop me to my knees. I didn't know what or when to eat, I couldn't sleep, and I was living on pain medication. That was very unlike me.

I eventually sought out the help of the old chiropractor. Keep in mind that in the 1970s, chiropractors were considered alternative practitioners. My chiropractor felt that I was suffering from a hiatal hernia, something that I had never heard of. In addition to treating me in his office, he taught me a self-massage technique, which over the course of a few weeks worked wonders.

That was many years before I went to school for my own chiropractic degree. Over the years, I've recommended this technique to a number of people who suffered from pain and heartburn for many years. Many of them, too, were amazed at the results they obtained.

SELF-MASSAGE TECHNIQUE FOR HIATAL HERNIA

While in a sitting position, locate your breastbone. It's that solid bone in the center of your body, between your breasts, connecting your ribs. It's below your throat and above your abdomen. Most people believe the heart is behind it. Another way to locate the breastbone is to place both your hands at the bottom of your ribcage and, following the bones of the ribcage, move them upwards and toward the center of your body. When you can't go any further, your fingers will be touching the base of your breastbone.

Move the tips of your fingers to an inch or so below the base of your breastbone. Now begin pressing your fingertips first up, then in, and then down. Up, in, and down. It's that simple. Using a constant rolling motion and a good amount of pressure, continue this self-massage for about one minute.

"Okay, big deal, now what?" you say. You're still feeling the same. Remember, this technique will require repetition over a period of about a week or two to bring results. Ultimately, you'll want to perform the self-massage for one full minute three or more times a day every day. But for the first several days, do the self-massage for just a few seconds once or twice a day.

Here's why. You perform the maneuver once or twice. The next day, you try it again, but you're probably unable to touch yourself comfortably. It feels like you're bruised, and you are. It's like going to the gym for the first time in a long time. Your muscle is sore and needs time to recover. (If you aren't bruised, you probably didn't push hard enough the first time.) Wait a day or two, then try it again. Within a few days, you should see your symptoms improving.

How does the technique work? A hernia is a section of stomach that has moved up and through the hole in the diaphragm, and the downward motion of the self-massage helps to pull it back down to its proper position. The upward motion of the maneuver puts your fingers in position to pull the tissue down.

CHIROPRACTIC-ASSISTED MANEUVER

For most hiatal hernias, the self-massage technique works very well. If it doesn't seem to bring you any relief, you might want to try a chiropractic-assisted maneuver.

Chiropractors have for years practiced an adjustment that brings the portion of the stomach extending up above the diaphragm back to its original position. The maneuver is very similar to the self-massage technique and frequently brings results in just one visit.

Even hiatal hernias can be treated better with a natural approach than with conventional medicine. Try the self-massage technique on your own for a few weeks and see what happens. If you feel you need professional help, find a chiropractor familiar with the chiropractic-assisted maneuver.

WHY DOESN'T MY DOCTOR KNOW THIS?

Conquering Irritable Bowel Syndrome, Inflammatory Bowel Disease, Crohn's Disease, and Colitis

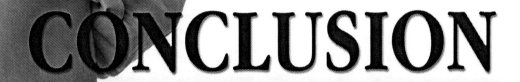

CONCLUSION

constipation

ulcers

blood

pain

gas

indigestion

spasms

heartburn

bloating

diarrhea

reflux

GERD

T he path to optimal health is yours to take alone. It is your responsibility. We can rely on others for their expertise, but at some point, our common sense must kick in and tell us there are answers we have not yet found.

I sincerely hope you have found the answers to your questions about your health concerns by reading about my all-natural protocol. You should now have a much better idea why you are experiencing your symptoms and what you should do about them. Though a simple statement—that it's all about bacteria and chemistry—rings throughout this book, determining what to do about these two issues can seem complex and confusing.

You now have learned how to reestablish a proper bacterial balance in your gastrointestinal system, and you have also read about the many ways you can affect your system's chemistry. The dietary considerations (no dairy, possibly no gluten and fructose) and the seemingly impossible rules based on your food allergy test results (if you needed to have that test) may seem daunting, but they are doable and they also are only temporary—or at least, most of them are temporary. Remember, many people have followed my protocol (and helped to fine-tune it), they were able to follow the rules and they were able to accomplish their goals. You can too.

As you attempt to navigate your way through the advice in this book, with or without the help of a physician, please remember to re-read certain parts of the program. The two that are the most important for carrying out the protocol properly are Chapter 5, "The Big Four Don't-You-Dare-Break-'Em Dietary Rules," and Chapter 6, "The Step-by-Step Thought Process." A less-than-full understanding of these two sections might be a recipe for failure. Take them seriously.

Though I hope all your questions have been answered, there is actually one I have done my best to answer but that may yet remain a mystery. The answer to that question, and the continued asking of the question, may well play an important role in moving healthcare to a more function-based, patient-centered place, making the elimination of chronic health conditions and the restoration of health using natural methods more accessible for everyone. That question is: *"Why didn't my doctor know this?"* Ask it as often as you can.

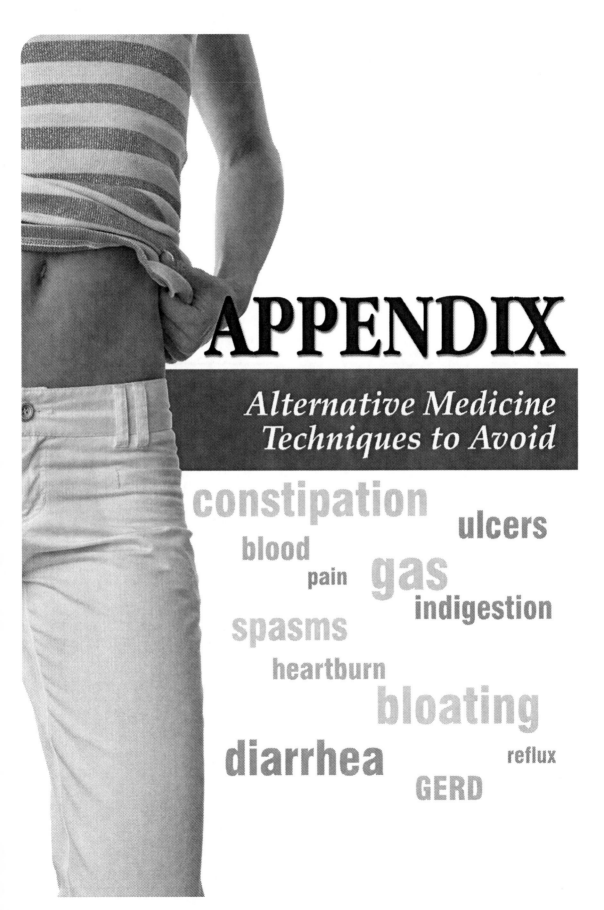

APPENDIX

Alternative Medicine Techniques to Avoid

constipation

ulcers

blood

pain

gas

indigestion

spasms

heartburn

bloating

diarrhea

reflux

GERD

It's funny how some people think that all alternative medicine is the same. I can't tell you how many times people have said to me that they've already tried alternative medicine as if there's only one protocol that's called "alternative medicine." Many people also think that what I would suggest for their condition is the same as what they've already tried. This is part of the problem with alternative medicine. My particular brand of alternative medicine falls into the category of holistic or nutritional medicine. While many other types of alternative medicine also fall into this category, not all do.

A better explanation is to call my form of alternative medicine "functional medicine." Simply put, it focuses on what is inhibiting the affected part or system of the body from functioning properly and what needs to be done to help it regain its function. It is based on the biochemical individuality of each patient, centered on patient care and not disease care, with an understanding that the human body is a network of interconnected systems, rather than individual systems functioning without effect on each other.

Once again, it needs to be said that the biggest failing of conventional medicine is its reliance on the principle that one simply needs to find one molecule to affect one process in the body to eliminate just one symptom. The body isn't that simple.

It is in this light that we take a look here at some of the other "therapies" that have been developed to help people overcome their gastrointestinal conditions. If you think you will find one product to help you overcome your IBS, then you need to *stop thinking like a conventional medical doctor!* Sorry for yelling.

I will also add that you need to be careful regarding any advice you receive. There are many people urging the use of treatments, pills, potions, herbs, vitamins, and such that worked for them. Gastrointestinal conditions are complex, as is the human body, and each patient is unique, so another person's success with a certain therapy doesn't guarantee that you will also see success, unless the approach is comprehensive.

In this appendix, we will examine some of the more common suggestions or treatments for gastrointestinal complaints and the reasons they may not work for you.

COLON HYDROTHERAPY

I get calls all the time from people looking for a colon hydrotherapist. I tell them how to find one if they insist, but I always ask why they would like to go to one. I'm usually given one of two answers. The first is that colon hydrotherapy was recommended either by a friend or by another doctor who didn't know what to do about IBS or constipation. The other answer is that they read something on the Internet or in a book about all the terrible creatures living inside the gut and/or about the fecal matter clinging to the walls of the intestines that can't possibly be removed any other way. They have determined that this must be the cause of their health problems.

What It Is

Colon hydrotherapy, also called a colonic, is the washing-out of the entire large intestine with a running source of water–sort of an enema on steroids. The device that's used has a Plexiglas window in the tube so the client can see what is coming out. The theory behind colon hydrotherapy is that the washing removes fecal matter stuck to the sides of the bowel, toxins, and parasites, and thereby improves the health.

Hydrotherapists add probiotics (acidophilus and *Bifidus*) to the water to help reestablish beneficial bacteria levels. They also add antiparasitic herbs to eliminate parasites. Most practitioners recommend return visits for a period of time. They also claim that they can see yeast being removed as they look at the content moving past the Plexiglas window.

The Reality

The truth is that colonics are unnecessary except in cases of impaction or constipation that doesn't respond to treatment. I can't remember the last time I had to make such a referral. The large intestine is a self-cleaning organ system. That's why we poop everyday.

The information on Web sites and in books touting colon hydrotherapy is incorrect. Fecal material rarely clings to the inside of the large intestine, unable to get out, putrefying and releasing toxins into the body. In cases of constipation, fecal material will release toxins, which are eventually reabsorbed into the system, but they are from fecal material sitting there during an abnormally long transit time, not from any material hanging there, attached to the wall of the colon.

Parasites are found in about 30 percent of the stool samples sent to labs across the country. These samples were taken from patients suspected of having the problem by a trained physician who specifically ordered the parasite test. I receive a finding of parasites in only one out of every 100 lab tests my office sends out each year. The herbs put in the water that washes out the colon are unnecessary. And the claim that the hydrotherapist can "see" yeast moving past the Plexiglas window ... well, yeast cannot be "seen" during a colonic. Yeast is a microscopic organism that can be identified only using a microscope in a lab.

The thought process behind colon hydrotherapy is also dangerous. If your main problem is constipation, and you find that a colonic relieves the uncomfortable full feeling and you use one every time you become uncomfortable, your bowel will lose the ability to function on its own. You can become as reliant on colonics as you can on laxatives. With both colonics and laxatives, the muscles attached to the bowel are not required to push the fecal material out because it's being artificially flushed out. Your bowels will never become balanced and learn to work properly on their own. This can result in your becoming stuck in a vicious cycle of experiencing constipation and then doing something repeatedly that never encourages your bowels to work on their own. Believe me, you don't have gastrointestinal problems because you don't have enough colonics!

Colon hydrotherapy is a technique that is at best simplistic in its approach. Washing out the large intestine doesn't reestablish proper levels of beneficial bacteria, even if probiotics (usually of poor quality and without the ability to remain in the intestines) are put in the water, and it doesn't restore the proper chemistry necessary for the health of the gastrointestinal system or figure out what foods are contributing to the problem. It doesn't wash out parasites or bacteria that shouldn't be living in the gastrointestinal tract. In other words, colon hydrotherapy at best might be a temporary fix, but it isn't a solution to the typical gastrointestinal complaints of people with IBS.

COLON CLEANSES

The concept of cleaning out your colon seems like a good idea. Who wouldn't want a clean colon? We just talked about colon hydrotherapy as a possible but not good answer. The manufacturers of colon cleanses, typically available in health food stores, over the Internet, and by direct mail, use similar scare tactics to get people to buy their products.

What It Is

The product packaging and advertisements for colon cleanses warn, again, that because of the fecal material tightly attached to the inside wall of your intestines and the parasites that live in it, you must use these products.

These products typically contain combinations of ingredients such as laxatives (senna, cascara sagrada), fiber (psyllium and others), bentonite (clay), and probiotics (acidophilus and *Bifidus*). Now, there is something to a treatment like this. You will have many bowel movements and feel as if you are cleaning out. Unfortunately, having a lot of bowel movements doesn't prove anything. Plus it has a downside.

The Reality

Many people who try colon cleanses end up with diarrhea because it's hard to regulate the amount of product to take to produce comfortable bowel movements. Most people wouldn't call going from constipation to diarrhea each day a benefit.

Other people report lots of gas and bloating, due to the fibers used in these products. And the probiotics in the products are usually worthless for a number of reasons, again primarily because they are poor quality and don't remain in the intestines. They will not help reestablish proper beneficial bacteria levels.

Colon cleanses don't reestablish proper bacterial balance or rid the gastrointestinal system of unwanted occupants. They also don't restore proper chemistry or point out offending foods. Again, they are at best a temporary fix, and they are not a solution to the typical gastrointestinal complaints of people with IBS.

HOMEOSTATIC SOIL ORGANISMS

Remember when Mom told you to stop eating dirt? It might have been good for you!

What It Is

Homeostatic soil organisms (HSOs) are beneficial bacteria (probiotics) usually found in soil. (I guess that's why they named them that.) Some people have found HSOs to be a useful product, as long as you don't mind a couple of problems.

The Reality

No specific strains of HSOs have been identified, and worse than that, you need to take them forever. They actually might help some with irritable bowel syndrome or any of the inflammatory bowel diseases. Until you stop taking them. The product's own directions suggest a larger dose for the first three months and then a smaller dose thereafter, with no suggestion of when you might be able to stop.

Once again, here is a product that doesn't reestablish proper bacterial levels, at least not permanently, or rid the gastrointestinal system of unwanted occupants. It also doesn't restore proper chemistry or point out offending foods. The same as the first two therapies we discussed, they are at best a temporary fix, and they are not a solution to the typical gastrointestinal complaints of people with IBS.

ALOE VERA

What It Is

Aloe vera has long been known as a healing substance. I used it in the early days of my practice to try to help people with irritable bowel syndrome. I prescribed aloe juice as a drink to take a couple of times each day. It was very helpful, although some of my office patients did experience side effects due to the anthraquinones in the aloe. My protocol has progressed by leaps and bounds since those days.

The Reality

The main aloe product on the market comes in tablet form and has had the anthraquinones removed. More than likely, this product does provide some benefit–until you stop taking it. Once again, the product's own directions suggest a larger dose initially, then a smaller dose, but no suggestion of when you might be able to stop.

So, now I'm beginning to sound like a broken record. Here is another product that doesn't reestablish proper bacterial levels, at least not permanently, or rid the gastrointestinal system of unwanted occupants. It doesn't restore proper chemistry or alert you to what foods might be contributing to your problem. Again, it might offer a temporary fix, but it isn't a solution to the typical gastrointestinal complaints of people with IBS.

MERACOL

What It Is

Meracol is the active ingredient in an Asian Pacific plant that contains fatty acid esters. Simply put, fatty acid esters are a derivative of the simple fats you eat everyday. Meracol is a specific ester from a plant that has been found to have anti-inflammatory properties and immune-enhancing abilities.

The Reality

Considering that the gastrointestinal system of people with irritable bowel syndrome or inflammatory bowel disease is probably inflamed and that 60 percent of a person's immune system operates there, Meracol can be expected to have beneficial effects. Until you stop taking it.

As usual with all the "easy" answers, the effects are temporary. Meracol also has a couple of other problems. If you are suffering from an inflammatory bowel disease such as Crohn's disease or any type of colitis, or from any other autoimmune condition, you can't use Meracol. Do you know if you've been properly diagnosed? What if your IBS is actually Crohn's disease or some type of colitis? If you're HIV positive or pregnant or a breastfeeding mother, you can't use it. If you have gallbladder disease or have had your gallbladder removed, you can't use it without an additional enzyme to help you digest the fats found in the product. Does this sound familiar to the advice I gave in Chapter 4 to people who have lost their gallbladder?

Here is another product that doesn't reestablish proper bacterial levels, at least not permanently, or rid the gastrointestinal system of unwanted occupants. It doesn't restore proper chemistry or alert you to what foods might be contributing to your problem. It might offer a temporary fix, but it isn't a solution to the typical gastrointestinal complaints of people with IBS.

SPECIFIC CARBOHYDRATE DIET

What It Is

Pioneered by Elaine Gottschall to rid her daughter of ulcerative colitis, this diet is the closest to the one presented in this book and was the first to put forth the concepts that dairy and gluten are among the potential villains in inflammatory bowel disease, irritable bowel syndrome, and celiac disease.

The Specific Carbohydrate Diet is based on the concept that all of the aforementioned conditions are due to imbalances in the microbial environment of the gastrointestinal system, and that the foods included in the diet have very specific chemistries that help restore the necessary balance. This protocol worked very well for Ms. Gottschall's daughter and has proven itself for thousands of others who have tried it. But I must warn that it doesn't work for everyone.

The Reality

The Specific Carbohydrate Diet has two potential shortcomings: It is both too restrictive and not comprehensive enough to address all the common gastrointestinal complaints.

First, it restricts foods that I have never, in fifteen years, required any of my patients to stop eating. It has all patients stop eating most dairy foods and all gluten-containing foods, but it also suggests not eating any rice or potatoes. I have found the elimination of rice and potatoes to be unnecessary for my patients unless we find through food allergy testing that they are allergic to them. Only a small percentage of patients do test allergic to them.

Second, it's not comprehensive enough when it comes to dairy being eliminated from the diet, and it does not call at all for a food allergy test. My protocol calls for the elimination of all dairy products. That's a 100-percent rule.

The Specific Carbohydrate Diet suggests eliminating all dairy products except fermented cheeses and a special yogurt that the author teaches how to make. The protocol is additionally lacking in terms of not recommending a food allergy test, as I have found it almost impossible to help people suffering from Crohn's disease or any type of colitis without such a test.

TREATMENTS FOR YEAST OVERGROWTH

What It Is

Many people call my office and say they believe they have an overgrowth of yeast based on a "test" they took that involved checking off all their symptoms and then scoring the results. If you have a high enough score, you are told you have a "systemic yeast" problem.

The Reality

An honest appraisal of the symptoms list in this "test" would make any rational person ask if there are any other possible symptoms a human could have that are not included on the list. The author of this "test" seems to believe that all symptoms are yeast related. This makes no sense to most people. So, don't rely on a test in a book or given to you at a health food store or by an "alternative" practitioner. Ask your physician for a laboratory test to check for the presence of yeast, and base your health decisions on objective findings.

The search for answers seems to be endless for people suffering from gastrointestinal conditions. Even temporary relief is welcome. I think we would all agree that permanent relief is what every sufferer is looking for. That should be the standard to which all treatments are held. If you are considering spending money on something that promises to solve IBS or an inflammatory bowel disease such as Crohn's disease or any type of colitis, simply ask one question: If I get relief from this product, what happens when I stop taking it?

For every product I know of on the market, the answer is that your symptoms may come back. As a sufferer, you know firsthand the frustration involved with these conditions. They are complex conditions requiring a complex plan of attack. Don't spend money month after month for relief that is just temporary. Instead, toss away the unproven supplements and therapies, and follow the protocol described in this book for a few months to end your suffering permanently.

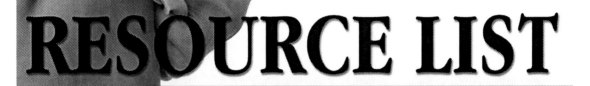

RESOURCE LIST

constipation

ulcers

blood

pain

gas

indigestion

spasms

heartburn

bloating

diarrhea

reflux

GERD

RESOURCE LIST

$\mathcal{T}$ he essential supplements (nutrients, herbs, and other compounds) I recommend in this book are all available from many sources. Below is the contact information for the five main suppliers I recommend. Some of these suppliers have the essential supplements available individually, while other sources have them mixed in with other nutrients as a combination product. Some do not carry the supplements we have discussed. Please note that you may not be able to match the essential supplements I use in my protocol with products from suppliers I do not use.

For the exact supplements used in Dr. Dahlman's protocol:

Dr. Dahlman's Online Store: www.drdahlman.meta-ehealth.com

2656 Fair Oaks Lane

Cincinnati, Ohio 45237

513-871-3300

info@drdahlman.com

www.drdahlman.com

Metagenics, Inc. (the supplier to Dr. Dahlman's Online Store)

100 Avenue La Pata

San Clemente, CA 92673

800-692-9400

www.metagenics.com

Other sources of similar supplements:

Allergy Research Group

2300 North Loop Road

Alameda, CA 94502

800-545-9960

info@allergyresearchgroup.com

www.allergyresearchgroup.com

PhytoPharmica, Inc.

825 Challenger Drive

Green Bay, WI 54311

800-376-7889

www.phytopharmica.com

Thorne Research, Inc.

25820 Highway 2 West

Sandpoint, ID 83864

208-263-1337

info@thorne.com

www.thorne.com

All the products listed below can be found from online sources by simply searching for the name of the recommended product on the Internet. All the products from PhytoPharmica can be found at most local health food stores.

RESOURCE LIST

ESSENTIAL SUPPLEMENTS TO REESTABLISH BACTERIAL BALANCE

Lactobacillus and Bifidobacterium

www.drdahlman.meta-ehealth.com

> LactoViden and BifoViden
>
>> –the exact supplements used by Dr. Dahlman

Allergy Research Group

> Symbiotics with FOS Powder
>
>> –a well thought out combination of *Lactobacillus, Bifidobacterium, Streptococcus thermophilus*, and FOS
>
> BifidoBiotics with L. sporogenes
>
>> –a good mix of Lactobacillus, Bifidobacterium, and FOS

Metagenics, Inc

> LactoViden and BifoViden
>
>> –the exact supplements used by Dr. Dahlman

PhytoPharmica

> Probiotic Pearls
>
>> –a low-dose, generic blend of *Lactobacillus and Bifidobacterium*

Thorne Research

> Lactobacillus Sporogenes
>
>> –a single-strain supplement

ESSENTIAL SUPPLEMENTS TO FEED TISSUE AND RESTORE CHEMISTRY

Rice Protein Powder

www.drdahlman.meta-ehealth.com

> UltraClear Sustain (also contains glutamine, other amino acids, inulin, and FOS)
>
> > —the exact supplement used by Dr. Dahlman

Metagenics, Inc

> UltraClear Sustain (also contains glutamine, other amino acids, inulin, and FOS)
>
> > —the exact supplement used by Dr. Dahlman

Thorne Research

> MediClear (also contains glutamine and other amino acids)
>
> > —a supplement very similar to that used by Dr. Dahlman

Glutamine

www.drdahlman.meta-ehealth.com

> UltraClear Sustain (also contains glutamine, other amino acids, inulin, and FOS)
>
> > —the exact supplement used by Dr. Dahlman
>
> Glutagenics
>
> > —a combination of glutamine, aloe, and licorice, for people with rice allergies

Allergy Research Group

> GastroCort II
>
> > —a glutamine supplement with additional synergistic compounds
>
> Perm-A-Vite
>
> > —a glutamine supplement with additional synergistic compounds

Metagenics, Inc

UltraClear Sustain (also contains glutamine, other amino acids, inulin, and FOS)

–the exact supplement used by Dr. Dahlman

Glutagenics

–a combination of glutamine, aloe, and licorice, for people with rice allergies

Thorne Research

MediClear

–a supplement very similar to that used by Dr. Dahlman

L-Glutamine Powder

–a supplement containing only glutamine

Other Amino Acids
N-acetylcysteine, L-glutathione, L-cysteine, L-lysine, and L-threonine

www.drdahlman.meta-ehealth.com

UltraClear Sustain (also contains glutamine, other amino acids, inulin, and FOS)

–the exact supplement used by Dr. Dahlman

Allergy Research Group

Free Aminos

–a blend of eighteen amino acids

L-glutamine

–a supplement containing only glutamine

L-Lysine

–a supplement containing only lysine

NAC

–a supplement containing only N-acetylcysteine

Metagenics, Inc

UltraClear Sustain (also contains glutamine, other amino acids, inulin, and FOS)

–the exact supplement used by Dr. Dahlman

Thorne Research

Cysteplus

–a supplement containing only N-acetylcysteine

Glutathione

–a supplement containing only glutathione

L-Lysine

–a supplement containing only lysine

Inulin

www.drdahlman.meta-ehealth.com

UltraClear Sustain (also contains glutamine, other amino acids, inulin, and FOS)

–the exact supplement used by Dr. Dahlman

Metagenics, Inc

UltraClear Sustain (also contains glutamine, other amino acids, inulin, and FOS)

–the exact supplement used by Dr. Dahlman

PhytoPharmica

Fiber Delights

–a blend of inulin and FOS

FOS (Fructo-oligosaccharides)

www.drdahlman.meta-ehealth.com

RESOURCE LIST

UltraClear Sustain (also contains glutamine, other amino acids, inulin, and FOS)

    –the exact supplement used by Dr. Dahlman

Allergy Research Group

    FOS Fructooligosaccharides

        –a supplement containing only FOS

Metagenics, Inc

    UltraClear Sustain (also contains glutamine, other amino acids, inulin, and FOS)

        –the exact supplement used by Dr. Dahlman

PhytoPharmica

    Fiber Delights

        –a blend of inulin and FOS

ESSENTIAL SUPPLEMENTS TO IMPROVE DIGESTION AND RESTORE pH

Betaine Hydrochloride, Pepsin, and Gentian Root

www.drdahlman.meta-ehealth.com

    Metagest

        –the exact supplement used by Dr. Dahlman

Allergy Reasearch Group

    Metaboliczyme

        –a broad-spectrum supplement for full digestion of proteins, carbs, and fat

Metagenics, Inc

> Metagest
>
> > —the exact supplement used by Dr. Dahlman

PhytoPharmica

> Pro-Gest
>
> > —a broad-spectrum supplement for full digestion of proteins, carbs, and fat

Thorne Research

> Betaine HCL/Pepsin
>
> > —a supplement containing betaine hydrochloride and pepsin

Protease, Amylase, and Lipase

www.drdahlman.meta-ehealth.com

> Azeo-Pangen
>
> > —the exact supplement used by Dr. Dahlman

Allergy Reasearch Group

> Metaboliczyme
>
> > —a broad-spectrum supplement for full digestion of proteins, carbs, and fat

Metagenics, Inc

> Azeo-Pangen
>
> > —the exact supplement used by Dr. Dahlman

RESOURCE LIST

PhytoPharmica

    CompleteGest

        –a vegetarian supplement for full digestion of proteins, carbs, and fat

    Bio-Zyme

        –a broad-spectrum supplement for full digestion of proteins, carbs, and fat

Thorne Research

    Dipan-9

        –a broad-spectrum supplement for full digestion of proteins, carbs, and fat

    Planti-Zyme

        –a vegetarian supplement for full digestion of proteins, carbs, and fat

Choline, Inositol, Taurine, and L-Methionine

www.drdahlman.meta-ehealth.com

    Lipo-Gen

        –the exact supplement used by Dr. Dahlman

Metagenics, Inc

    Lipo-Gen

        –the exact supplement used by Dr. Dahlman

Thorne Research

    Lipotrepein

        –a blend containing choline, inositol, taurine, methionine, and other
synergistic compounds

Peppermint, Chamomile, and Lavender Oils

www.drdahlman.meta-ehealth.com

    Intesol

        –the exact supplement used by Dr. Dahlman

Metagenics, Inc

    Intesol

        –the exact supplement used by Dr. Dahlman

PhytoPharmica

    Mentharil

        –a supplement containing peppermint, rosemary, and thyme

ANTI-ANAEROBIC BACTERIAL SUPPLEMENTS

Coptis Root, Indian Barberry, and Berberine

www.drdahlman.meta-ehealth.com

    Candibactin BR and Ulcinex

        –the exact supplements used by Dr. Dahlman

Allergy Reasearch Group

    Tricycline

        –a combination supplement containing berberine, artemisinin, citrus

        seed, and black walnut

RESOURCE LIST

Metagenics, Inc

    Candibactin BR and Ulcinex

        –the exact supplements used by Dr. Dahlman

PhytoPharmica

    Berberine Complex

        –a combination of berberine and goldenseal

Thorne Research

    Coptis

        –a supplement containing coptis

    Berbercap

        –a supplement containing berberine and coptis

PEPTIC ULCER DISEASE SUPPLEMENT (ZINC CARNOSINE)

www.drdahlman.meta-ehealth.com

    Zinlori 75

        –the exact supplement used by Dr. Dahlman

Metagenics, Inc

    Zinlori 75

        –the exact supplement used by Dr. Dahlman

Note: Many health food stores carry a product that is similar but that has a lower dose than the 75 milligrams proven in studies to be the most effective.

ANTI-INFLAMMATORY SUPPLEMENTS

Ginger, Tumeric, Citruline, D-limonene, Rosemary Leaf, Hesperidine, Rutin, and Quercetin

www.drdahlman.meta-ehealth.com

UltraInflamX 360 Plus (also contains glutamine, ginger, tumeric, citruline, d-limonene, rosemary leaf, hesperidine, rutin, and quercetin)

–the exact supplement used by Dr. Dahlman

Inflavonoid Intensive Care

–a supplement containing ginger, tumeric, citruline, d-limonene, rosemary leaf, hesperidine, rutin, and quercetin

Metagenics, Inc

UltraInflamX 360 Plus (also contains glutamine, ginger, tumeric, citruline, d-limonene, rosemary leaf, hesperidine, rutin, and quercetin)

–the exact supplement used by Dr. Dahlman

Inflavonoid Intensive Care

–a supplement containing ginger, tumeric, citruline, d-limonene, rosemary leaf, hesperidine, rutin, and quercetin

PhytoPharmica

AlzClear

–a supplement containing tumeric

GingerMax

–a supplement containing ginger

RESOURCE LIST

Thorne Research

    Phytoprofen

        –a supplement containing boswelia and tumeric

    Curcumin

        –a supplement containing curcumin

    Quercetone

        –a supplement containing quercetin

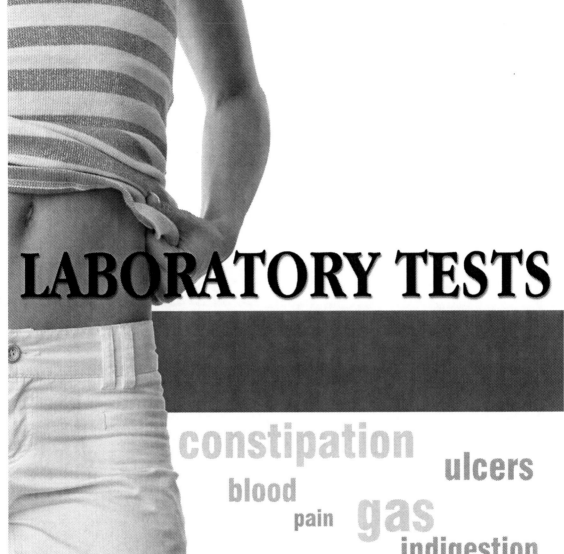

LABORATORY TESTS

constipation

ulcers

blood

pain

gas

indigestion

spasms

heartburn

bloating

diarrhea

reflux

GERD

LABORATORY TESTS

Isn't it amazing to think that even though the typical IBS or inflammatory bowel disease patient has been tested up this way and down that way, there could be some additional tests that would be more useful? Has your doctor ordered stool or food allergy testing? Depending on the lab your doctor ordered the test from, it may not be complete enough to provide you with information that will contribute to your recovery. Additionally, your doctor may be looking in the wrong place. Confused?

Rarely do the typical tests that people with gastrointestinal complaints endure–such as a colonoscopy, endoscopy, barium enema, acid production test, CAT scan, or MRI–yield the reason for their symptoms. This doesn't mean you shouldn't have the test. It might save your life from a more serious condition. But it rarely finds the cause of your gastrointestinal complaints. And there's a lot to be said for the peace of mind you get when you learn there's nothing seriously wrong with you.

If your doctor orders a stool test, you trust his or her judgment, but exactly what is the doctor testing for? Is the test just for parasites? Does it include a look at the bacterial balances? If it looks at the bacterial balances, does this include the levels of both the good and the bad bacteria? Were you tested for the presence of a yeast overgrowth? The right test must be ordered from the right lab, looking for the right organisms, or you may not get any useful information. Once again, you run the risk of leaving your doctor's office feeling empty and still with no answers.

Many labs offer the same or similar tests, and more than likely, if your doctor has ordered the tests from a local independent lab or a local hospital, the results will be incomplete. If you returned a stool sample to your doctor's office or had your blood drawn there, you can be sure that the sample went to the wrong lab. There are labs around the country whose specialty is looking at the testing needs of doctors who are committed to finding the causes of patients' problems (patient-centered care) and design their tests from a completely different perspective.

I have found that approximately a third of my patients reach a point in my program where they need laboratory testing. If you go back to Chapter 6, "The Step-by-Step Thought Process," you will read about when I suggest a person undergo stool and food allergy tests, the two main tests that help people with IBS. You should know that although a food allergy test can provide valuable information for anyone, not many people ever need that test. Let me make the point that if a person has been diagnosed with any form of colitis or Crohn's disease, the food allergy test will be the first test conducted at the beginning of my protocol. (See Chapter 9, "Crohn's Disease and Any Type of Colitis.")

The laboratory I use for both stool and food allergy testing is Genova Diagnostics Laboratory in Asheville, North Carolina. This lab used to be known as Great Smokies Diagnostic Laboratory. The descriptions I use in this section are about the tests from this lab, but all stool and allergy testing is similar, so it should not be difficult to pick tests from other labs and interpret the results in the same manner I describe here if you wish not to use Genova.

Genova Diagnostics

63 Zillicoa Street

Asheville, NC 28801

800-522-4762

www.GDX.net

There are many other labs across the country that conduct similar tests, such as:

Great Plains Laboratory (food allergy and stool tests)

11813 West 77th Street

Lenexa, KS 66214

913-341-8949

www.greatplainslaboratory.com

LABORATORY TESTS

Immunosciences Lab, Inc. (food allergy and stool tests)

8693 Wilshire Boulevard

Suite 200

Beverly Hills, CA 90211

800-950-4686

www.immuno-sci-lab.com

Meta Metrix Clinical Lab (food allergy tests)

4855 Peachtree Industrial Blvd

Suite 201

Norcross, GA 30092

800-221-4640

www.metametrix.com

U.S. Bio Tek Laboratories (food allergy tests)

13500 Linden Avenue North

Seattle, WA 98133

206-365-1256

www.usbiotek.com

All of the following tests are available through your doctor. The discussions include what the tests are for, when to use them, how to interpret the findings, and what products to use to bring the results into normal ranges.

Stool Testing

Bacteria and Yeast Testing

Purpose. The purpose of this test is to provide information about normal and abnormal bacteria and yeast currently in the patient's gastrointestinal tract. Abnormal levels of either good or bad organisms can be detrimental to overall health and contribute to symptoms. It's the most common test used in my office. The good bacteria of most concern are *Lactobacillus acidophilus* and *Bifidobacterium*, which are also known as acidophilus and *Bifidus*, respectively. This test also names any potentially bad bacteria or yeast organisms, also known as candida or fungal organisms (that's right–technically they are a fungus), that might be living inside the gut. Each organism is named, and the amount found is noted (see "How to Interpret," below).

When to Use. If you refer back to Chapter 6, "The Step-by-Step Thought Process," and re-read Step Three, you'll see I use this test when a patient experiences additional gas and bloating within the first day or two after beginning my program. This additional gas and bloating is the number-one clinical indicator that identifies the need for this test. Remember my story about feeding the bad bacteria as being the cause of additional gas and bloating?

How to Interpret. What my experience has shown is that if a patient needs to take this test because of additional gas and bloating, we will probably find information that will be helpful in the elimination of symptoms. The test has three headings, with lab findings under each one.

Beneficial Bacteria. This section of the test lists the two most important strains of bacteria that we want to be at optimal levels–acidophilus and *Bifidus*. The test ranks their populations, using bar graphs next to the names of the bacteria, on a scale from NG (no growth) to 4+. These numbers are placed on the bar graph with corresponding colors. Optimal levels are achieved at the 3+ and 4+ levels, and should be in a white area. Anything under 3+ or 4+ needs to be addressed with the probiotic supplements described in Chapter 4 until optimal levels are reached. The test also reports the level of *Eschieria coli (E. coli)*, a normal part of bowel flora. No matter what level of *E. coli* is reported, nothing can be done to change it. If the level is too low, it may rise on its own after all the other bacterial levels are successfully restored.

Abnormal Bacteria. In this section, the test lists any other bacteria found and ranks their populations using the same bar graph and scale as for the beneficial bacteria. The numbers are also placed in colored areas. However, different colors (yellow and red) are used, and another criterion is included–a box next to the name of the organism describes whether it's nonpathogenic (NP), possibly pathogenic (PP), or pathogenic (P). You will find the numbers for a possible pathogen (PP) placed in a section of the bar graph colored yellow and for a pathogen (P) in a section of the graph colored red. The word "pathogen" means that the little critter, in the amounts found, can cause problems. If the information states it is a possible pathogen (PP) or a pathogen (P), treatment is needed to eliminate the organism so that the beneficial bacteria can grow to optimal levels. Remember, that was our original intent in this whole process.

As with the beneficial bacteria, there usually are some bacteria reported here that can be ignored. Some that might be mentioned are alpha or gamma haemolytic *Streptococcus* or coagulase negative *Staphylococcus*, which are nonpathogenic (NP) and placed in a white area of the bar graph. Don't worry about them.

There is one additional situation that requires some interpretation, or, shall we say, some clinical decision making. It is possible that additional bacteria will be listed here as nonpathogenic (NP) and not in a colored area, yet might still be a potential problem. They can have many different names that a trained physician familiar with this test will recognize but that mean nothing to you. You may find two or three of them in amounts of 1+ or 2+. Let's say there are two organisms listed as nonpathogenic (NP) and 2+. The laboratory has standard guidelines when it comes to reporting findings, so it must list each individual organism and its possibility for being a pathogen without regard to what it is and without regard to the other organisms found. So, we have two organisms listed as 2+. Well, I make the decision that 2+ plus 2+ equals 4+, and any one organism at a 4+ would be listed as a pathogen (P). So, is it possible that these two organisms, though lower in amounts individually, cumulatively equate to what one organism would be at a higher amount? My experience says yes, and I treat the person as if these two organisms in tandem are a pathogen (P) and get rid of both of them.

Yeast. This is the section that reports the findings concerning yeast. The organisms found are reported using the same bar graph, scale, color system, and designation as nonpathogenic (NP), possibly pathogenic (PP), or pathogenic (P) as abnormal bacteria. Again, it is possible, as with the abnormal bacteria, for you to have two types of yeast organism that are listed as nonpathogenic (NP) but, because of their cumulative effect, will still need to be treated as if they were pathogenic (P).

Sensitivities and Product Usage. A valuable part of this test report is the sensitivity section because it tells the doctor what to use to eliminate any abnormal organisms. When lab technicians find abnormal bacteria or yeast in a patient's sample, they grow it in the lab and then apply all-natural herbal remedies, other all-natural compounds, and prescription medications to see which products kill the organism. They then report which products were the most effective. This section of the report also utilizes a bar graph, to rank the products according to their ability to kill the organism. Three columns with bar graphs describe how the organism reacted to each product–most sensitive (S), intermediate sensitivity (I), or resistant (R). It is best to use the products that have the bar graph extending under the S, for most sensitive.

All patients have the option of using either all-natural products or prescription medication. Most patients opt for the all-natural products. The typical natural products used are berberine, uva ursi, garlic, plant tannins, oregano, and undecenoic acid (a derivative of the castor bean), all available at local health food stores. A one-month course of treatment is often, but not always, enough to kill any abnormal findings.

Retest needed? Absolutely. Any doctor who treated a patient for the findings of a stool test and doesn't retest is doing the patient a disservice whether a prescription medication or a natural compound was used to eliminate the abnormal findings of the test. How would we know if the treatment was effective? It would be impossible if we didn't retest. After the one-month treatment, send another sample to the lab. But for which test?

❖ If in the first test you had abnormal findings for both abnormal bacteria and yeast, retest for both.

❖ If you had abnormal findings only for abnormal bacteria, retest for just the abnormal findings using bacteria testing (see below).

❖ If you had abnormal findings only for yeast, test for just yeast using yeast testing (see below).

❖ If you had abnormal findings only for beneficial bacteria, retest for just beneficial bacteria using bacteria testing (see below).

Bacteria Testing

Purpose. The purpose of this test is to provide information about normal and abnormal bacteria currently in the patient's gastrointestinal tract. Abnormal levels of either good or bad organisms can be detrimental to overall health and contribute to symptoms. The good bacteria of most concern are *Lactobacillus acidophilus* and *Bifidobacterium*, which are also known as acidophilus and *Bifidus*, respectively. This test also names any potentially bad bacteria that might be living inside the gut. Each organism is named, and the amount found is noted (see "How to Interpret," below).

When to Use. This test is never used as the first test for a patient. It is usually used to retest a patient who has undergone treatment for the abnormal findings of a bacteria and yeast test.

How to Interpret.

The test has two headings, with lab findings under each one.

Beneficial Bacteria. This section of the test lists the two most important strains of bacteria that we want to be at optimal levels–acidophilus and Bifidus. The test ranks their populations, using bar graphs next to the names of the bacteria, on a scale from NG (no growth) to 4+. These numbers are placed on the bar graph with corresponding colors. Optimal levels are achieved at the 3+ and 4+ levels, and should be in a white area. Anything under 3+ or 4+ needs to be addressed with the probiotic supplements described in Chapter 4 until optimal levels are reached. The test also reports the level of *Eschieria coli (E. coli)* , a normal part of bowel flora. No matter what level of *E. coli* is reported, nothing can be done to change it. If the level is too low, it may rise on its own after all the other bacterial levels are successfully restored.

Abnormal Bacteria. In this section, the test lists any other bacteria found and ranks their populations using the same bar graph and scale as for the beneficial bacteria. The numbers are also placed in colored areas. However, different colors (yellow and red) are used, and another criterion is included–a box next to the name of the organism describes whether it's nonpathogenic (NP), possibly pathogenic (PP), or pathogenic (P). The word "pathogen" means that the

Controversy About "Normal" Bacterial Levels

Many times, patients will show the results from a stool test requested by another physician to their current physician and get a response that surprises them. Some physicians may feel that the strains of bacteria the lab identified as "abnormal" are not abnormal at all. In fact, they may believe these strains of bacteria are normal in a healthy human gastrointestinal system.

To some degree they are right, except that what they fail to notice is that the test results identify the amounts of these organisms and what is abnormal is not that they are present, but that the organisms are present in such high amounts. If their amounts were reduced, their negative effects on the gastrointestinal system and their contributions to the person's symptoms would go away. They would still be present in the gastrointestinal tract, just not in as high a number.

Don't let your physician dismiss your concerns about test results.

Let's Kill the Yeast Diet

In addition to using all-natural supplements to kill yeast organisms, you also need to starve the little critters of their favorite foods. Yeast organisms seem to thrive on certain foods. During the time you use the all-natural supplements to eliminate their overgrowth, you also need to follow a specific diet. You will fail to eliminate the yeast organisms from your gut if you don't first eliminate from your diet the foods that nourish them.

There are many variations of the anti-yeast diet. The rules you are about to read are the simplest combination that I have found to be effective. The basic program in this book takes away so many foods, albeit hopefully temporarily, that I try to eliminate as few as possible to get the best results. Don't despair. This is just for now, just for the next month, while you take your all-natural supplements. As soon as a retest indicates your yeast levels have returned to normal, you can forget about these rules.

The foods you must stay away from are all fruits, anything sweetened with added sugar (you must lose your sweet tooth), all gluten-containing foods, all fermented foods, and all foods made with or containing yeast.

Why did you develop a yeast overgrowth? The candida organism is a normal part of the human gastrointestinal system. Let's think back to my original premise. Antibiotics are the primary--not the only, but the primary--reason that the beneficial bacteria levels are altered in the gut. Antibiotics are designed to kill bacteria, but not yeast. Yeast is a fungus and needs an antifungal to kill it.

If you take an antibiotic that alters the amount of bacteria in your gastrointestinal system, there will be some vacant real estate down there. The yeast will therefore overgrow because they are not being held in check by the bacterial population. This is the same reason women get vaginal yeast infections after taking antibiotics. All mucosal membranes in the body have a bacterial-fungal balance. Vaginally, if a woman takes an antibiotic, the normal flora of her vagina is altered and the yeast are able to reproduce to abnormal levels because they're not limited by the bacterial levels. The woman must then take an antifungal pill or apply an antifungal cream to return her yeast population to normal so her beneficial bacteria levels can rise once again.

Quick tip: A way to avoid a vaginal yeast infection after taking a course of antibiotics is to take beneficial bacteria orally or to douche with them. Use the essential supplements to reestablish beneficial bacteria discussed in Chapter 4. Put one teaspoon of acidophilus and *Bifidus* into water, and douche with this formula in the morning and again at bedtime for a couple of days. You can use a bit less and do this every day you're on the antibiotic, then for a couple of days after you're done. There's no exact way; it's an individual call. Figure out what works best for you.

little critter, in the amounts found, can cause problems. If the information states it is a possible pathogen (PP) or a pathogen (P), treatment is needed to eliminate the organism so that the beneficial bacteria can grow to optimal levels. Remember, that was our original intent in this whole process.

As with the beneficial bacteria, there usually are some bacteria reported here that can be ignored. Some that might be mentioned are alpha or gamma haemolytic *Streptococcus* or coagulase negative *Staphylococcus*, which are nonpathogenic (NP) and placed in a white area of the bar graph. Don't worry about them.

There is one additional situation that requires some interpretation, or, shall we say, some clinical decision making. It is possible that additional bacteria will be listed here as nonpathogenic (NP) and not in a colored area, yet might still be a potential problem. They can have many different names that a trained physician familiar with this test will recognize but that mean nothing to you. You may find two or three of them in amounts of 1+ or 2+. Let's say that there are two organisms listed as nonpathogenic (NP) and 2+. The laboratory has standard guidelines when it comes to reporting findings, so it must list each individual organism and its possibility for being a pathogen without regard to what it is. So, we have two organisms listed as 2+. Well, I make the decision that 2+ plus 2+ equals 4+, and any one organism at a 4+ would be listed as a pathogen (P). So, is it possible that these two organisms, though lower in amounts individually, cumulatively equate to what one organism would be at a higher amount? My experience says yes, and I treat the person as if these two organisms in tandem are a pathogen (P) and get rid of both of them.

Sensitivities and Product Usage. A valuable part of this test report is the sensitivity section because it tells the doctor what to use to eliminate any abnormal organisms. When lab technicians find abnormal bacteria in a patient's sample, they grow it in the lab and then apply all-natural herbal remedies, other all-natural compounds, and prescription medications to see which products kill the organism. They then report which products were the most effective. This section of the report also utilizes a bar graph, to rank the products according to their ability to kill the organism. Three columns with bar graphs describe how the organism reacted to each product–most sensitive (S), intermediate sensitivity (I), and resistant (R). It is best to use the products that have the bar graph extending under the S.

All patients have the option of using either all-natural products or prescription medication. Most patients opt for the all-natural products. The typical natural products used are berberine, uva ursi, garlic, plant tannins, and oregano, all available at local health food stores. A one-month course of treatment is often, but not always, enough to kill any abnormal findings.

Retest needed? Maybe. If all the parameters in the retest are normal, a second retest will not be needed. However, if the retest continues to show abnormal findings for either beneficial bacteria or abnormal bacteria, resume treatment for another month, this time following the recommendations of the new report, and then retest again.

Yeast Testing

Purpose. The purpose of this test is to provide information about the yeast levels currently in the patient's gastrointestinal tract. Abnormal levels of yeast, also known as candida, can be detrimental to overall health and contribute to symptoms. This test also specifies exactly which types of yeast organisms are living inside the patient. Each organism is named, and the amount found is noted (see "How to Interpret," below).

When to Use. This test is never used as the first test for a patient. It is usually used to retest a patient who has undergone treatment for the abnormal findings of a bacteria and yeast test.

How to Interpret.

This test has one heading, with lab findings underneath.

Mycology. This section of the test reports findings of yeast. The test ranks the populations of the different types, using bar graphs next to their names, on a scale from NG (no growth) to 4+. These numbers are placed on the bar graph with corresponding colors. In addition, a box next to the name of the organism describes whether it's nonpathogenic (NP), possibly pathogenic (PP), or pathogenic (P). You will find the numbers for a possible pathogen (PP) placed in a section of the bar graph colored yellow and for a pathogen (P) in a section of the graph colored red. The word "pathogen" means that the little critter, in the amounts found, can cause problems. If the information states it is a possible pathogen (PP) or a pathogen (P), treatment is needed to eliminate the organism so that the beneficial bacteria can grow to optimal levels. Remember, that was our original intent in this whole process. Note that it is also possible that two different types of yeast may individually be listed as nonpathogenic (NP) but, because of their cumulative effects, will need to be treated as if they were pathogenic (P).

Sensitivities and Product Usage. A valuable part of this test report is the sensitivity section because it tells the doctor what to use to eliminate any abnormal organisms. When lab technicians find abnormal yeast in a patient's sample, they grow it in the lab and then apply all-natural herbal remedies, other all-natural compounds, and prescription medications to see which products kill the organism. They then report which products were the most effective. This section of the report also utilizes a bar graph, to rank the products according to their ability to kill the organism. Three columns with bar graphs describe how the organism reacted to each product—most sensitive (S), intermediate sensitivity (I), or resistant (R). It is best to use the products that have the bar graph extending under the S, for most sensitive.

All patients have the option of using either all-natural products or prescription medication. Most patients opt for the all-natural products. The typical natural products used are berberine, garlic, undecenoic acid (a derivative of the castor bean), plant tannins, and uva ursi, all available at local health food stores. A one-month course of treatment is often, but not always, enough to kill any abnormal findings.

Note: Not only do you need to use products to kill the yeast organisms, but you must also starve them of the foods they love. This two-pronged approach is the key to elimination of these organisms. If you use only an all-natural or prescription product and do not eliminate the problem foods, your chances for success will be greatly reduced. For dietary guidelines, please read "The Let's Kill the Yeast Diet" and add its rules to the Big Four Don't-You-*Dare*-Break-'Em Dietary Rules, which you are already following. Yeah, I know we're running out of foods choices, but you can do this!

Retest needed? Maybe. If all the parameters in the retest are normal, a second retest will not be needed. However, if the retest continues to show abnormal findings for yeast, resume treatment for another month, this time following the recommendations of the new report, and then retest again.

Parasite Testing

Purpose. The purpose of this test is to identify the presence of any parasites. I have left this discussion for the last because very few patients will need this test. Parasites are rarely found in patients complaining of gastrointestinal complaints. I might see one out of 100 each year.

When to Use. If you have navigated your way through Chapter 6, "The Step-by-Step Thought Process," and are still having symptoms, consider having this test, as it may reveal a problem. You should also consider taking it if you have traveled to a Third World country, lived on or visited a farm, or swam in a creek or stream, or have any other reason to suspect you might have picked up a parasite.

How to Interpret.

Interpretation is easy. You either have a parasite or you do not.

Sensitivities and Product Usage. The most effective treatment will be a prescription medication based on the type of parasite found. Natural treatment may also be effective and could include the use of herbs such as goldenseal, garlic, artemisia (wormwood), bitterwood, black walnut, and oil of oregano.

Food Allergy Testing

Purpose

In my office, food allergy testing is used as a final diagnostic tool for a small percentage of patients being treated for IBS and as a first diagnostic tool for all patients being treated for inflammatory bowel disease, Crohn's disease, or any type of colitis. Food allergies can create an immune response that affects the gastrointestinal system, making the test extremely important.

Using a blood sample, the laboratory will test for immunoglobulin G (IgG) reactions to eighty-eight common foods using an ELISA laboratory protocol. This is quite a different test than the conventional skin-prick test. There are two types of reactions a person can have to foods–immediate sensitivity, which is mediated by immunoglobulin E (IgE), and delayed sensitivity, mediated by IgG. Immediate (IgE) reactions are responsible for the symptoms associated with the reactions to well-known allergens such as peanuts, shellfish, and soy. People know when they have a reaction like that as they get symptoms quickly. In some cases, they are also responsible for the uncomfortable symptoms people get from eating foods to which they are sensitive but not allergic.

IgG reactions, since they are delayed, can be identified only through laboratory testing. A delayed response by the immune system results from the creation of a number of chemicals that have many different effects throughout the body, but especially from histamine. This is the only immune system response that interests me because these are the allergies that patients cannot figure out on their own (see Chapter 7, "Why You Have Other Health Complaints").

Delayed reactions are important and explain why intelligent people who pay close attention to their body and its reactions to food can't figure out which foods are truly causing their problems. Many patients, given enough time, throw their hands up and begin to eat hardly anything.

LABORATORY TESTS

When you can eat something on Tuesday for lunch and not have a reaction to it until Thursday evening, it's no wonder you can't tie the two events together and identify the food involved.

There are two different types of testing protocols used by laboratories—RAST (radioallergosorbent) and ELISA (enzyme-linked immunosorbent assay). RAST is used for immediate sensitivities, and ELISA is used for both immediate and delayed sensitivities.

A skin-prick test using RAST is known for being highly inaccurate because of a high number of false positives and false negatives. The ELISA test, which looks for the actual antibody that has been produced in the bloodstream, is far more reliable, although still not perfect.

When to Use

Please refer to Chapter 6, "The Step-By-Step Thought Process," Step 7, if you have IBS and Chapter 9, "Crohn's Disease and Any Type of Colitis," if you have an inflammatory bowel disease to learn when you should have a food allergy test.

How to Interpret

Interpretation is actually very simple. Refer immediately to the summary of the findings. The foods for which you were tested will be ranked according to the severity of your reaction to them. One rating system uses 3+, 2+, 1+, VL (very low), and zero. Though the instructions you receive from the lab may say otherwise, the only foods you should eat for the next six months will be ranked under the zero. All foods in the 3+, 2+, 1+, and VL categories must be avoided or you may not get the results you are looking for. There is controversy within the medical community over how long you must avoid a food to get rid of an allergy to it. The range is from twenty-eight days to six months. I believe in erring on the side of the conservative and shooting for the six-month mark.

When looking at the summarized test results, pay attention not only to the foods you are allergic to and must avoid, but also to the list of foods you are not allergic to. This latter list is the list of foods you are allowed to eat. If a food is not on the list of foods you are not allergic to, do not eat it. The reason for this is that there are more foods available than the common ones the lab chooses to test for. Therefore, if you were not tested for a certain food, you won't know if you are allergic to it or not. For example, if you love cantaloupe and eat it frequently but your lab's food panel didn't include it, don't eat it, since you won't have any data about it.

Also, once you have a list of foods you are not allergic to, if you have IBS, you should cross out any dairy products and continue to avoid them. Crohn's disease and colitis patients should cross out all dairy products as well as all gluten-containing foods. Please remember that this test looks for food allergies, not food intolerances. Because of suspected intolerances to these food groups, I remove all dairy products at the beginning of my IBS protocol and all dairy and gluten-containing foods at the beginning of my IBD protocol. Please review my discussion of this topic in Chapter 6, "The Step-by-Step Thought Process."

Many labs provide a suggested schedule for reintroducing foods into the diet. Throw it away, as it will only confuse you and cause you to not see the results you are looking for. Stay away from the foods that you have been found to have any level of reaction to, and do so for a minimum of six months. Then, conservatively reintroduce these foods without overeating any of them. There's no science to it; just eat a few of them each day, and rotate them throughout the week. Make it simple.

Laboratory testing can be the key that opens up the lock that guards the answers you are seeking. For many people, it isn't enough to take some supplements and stay away from a few foods or food groups. Objective diagnostic testing is just as and sometimes more important. To successfully reestablish your beneficial bacteria balances, you may need to have a stool test to identify any unwelcome critters that might be living in your gut. In addition, food allergy testing can fine-tune your food eliminations. Both types of tests can identify specific problems that when left unidentified can keep you running around chasing your tail in frustration. Find a doctor who is willing to use these tests and who understands them.

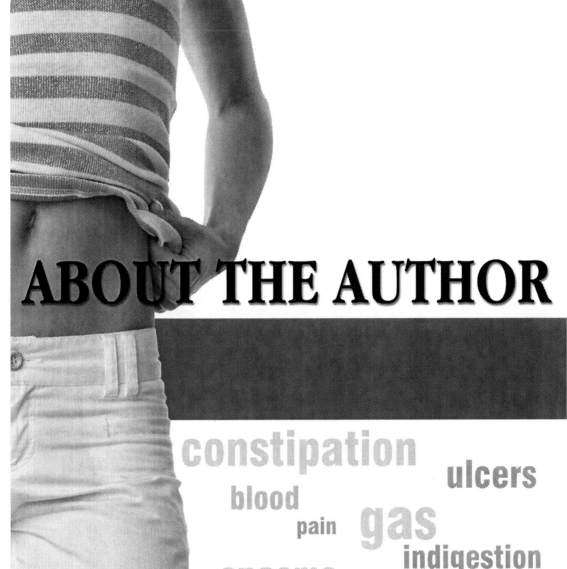

ABOUT THE AUTHOR

constipation

ulcers

blood

pain

gas

indigestion

spasms

heartburn

bloating

diarrhea

reflux

GERD

ABOUT THE AUTHOR

David Dahlman, DC is a chiropractic physician with a degree in nutrition. As Director of the Hyde Park Holistic Center in Cincinnati, Ohio, he has specialized in the treatment of chronic health conditions using nutritional, herbal and alternative therapies since the early 1990's.

His experience with more than 10,000 patients has lead him to develop all natural treatment protocols for a wide variety of chronic health conditions such as IBS, Crohn's Disease, Colitis, arthritis, Fibromyalgia, allergies, headaches, adrenal and thyroid conditions, female hormone imbalances, heart disease, diabetes and others.

Regardless of the challenge or condition presented, his treatment protocols have always focused on the gastrointestinal system and its influence on human health.

In his ongoing efforts to promote a healthy lifestyle, he is the past publisher of ***The Cincinnati Natural Resource Guide: A Guide to Health, Wellness and Environmental Products and Services.*** He also has experience as a weekly columnist for *CityBeat Magazine*, an alternative weekly published in the Greater Cincinnati area as well as host of a weekly radio health talk show on 55KRC in Cincinnati.

Dr. Dahlman has enjoyed and professed a healthful diet for more than 30 years. He has participated in more than 100 triathlons, duathlons and marathons in the U.S. and Europe since the 1980's.

His main focus is to educate the public that they have natural alternatives that address the cause of their condition as opposed to conventional medical treatments that only suppress symptoms.

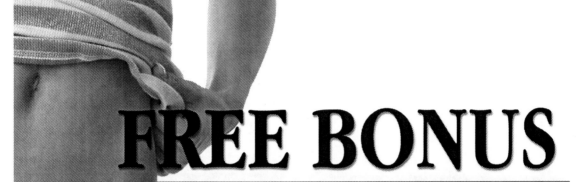

FREE BONUS

constipation
ulcers
blood
pain
gas
indigestion
spasms
heartburn
bloating
diarrhea
reflux
GERD

FREE BONUS

Because of the trust you have placed in me by purchasing this book, I would like to thank you and offer some additional valuable information. I want you to take full advantage of the information I have presented to help you conquer IBS, Crohn's Disease or any form of colitis..... so,

What I have prepared for you is a Video Consultation on DVD that I am planning on making available to the public in the near future. I would like you to have it first. It will summarize the key points important for your recovery and also describe for you the **EXACT** supplement program I use for the patients in my office. I name names and also dosages of the exact supplements I use that have resulted in the elimination of the symptoms of IBS, Crohn's Disease and any form of colitis for almost every one of my patients.

To view this information, please go to:

www.WhyDoesn'tMyDoctorKnowThis.com

You can view the DVD as video on my website and learn the names of the exact supplements, the dosages I recommend and the easiest way to purchase them...and you can go back time after time to review the material.

Thanks so much for your trust in me and my protocol. Here's to your health!

REFERENCES

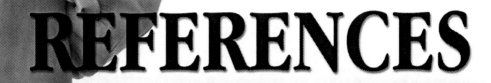

constipation

ulcers

blood

pain

gas

indigestion

spasms

heartburn

bloating

diarrhea

reflux

GERD

REFERENCES

Abela MB. Hypnotherapy for Crohn's disease: a promising complementary/alternative therapy. Integr Med 2000;2(2/3):127–131.

Adewunni CO, Oguntimein BO, Furu P. Molluscicidal and antischistosomal activities of Zingiber officinale. Planta Med 1990;36:374–76.

Agnihotri S, Vaidya ADB. A novel approach to study antibacterial properties of volatile components of selected Indian medicinal herbs. Indian J Exp Biol 1996;34:712–15.

Ajello M, Greco R, Giansanti F, et al. Anti-invasive activity of bovine lactoferrin towards group A streptococci. Biochem Cell Biol 2002;80(1):119–24.

Alic M. Green tea for remission maintenance in Crohn's disease? Am J Gastroenterol. 1999;94(6):1710

Anand BS, Romero JJ, Sanduja SK, et al. Phospholipid association reduces the gastric mucosal toxicity of aspirin in human subjects. Am Coll Gastroenterol 1999;94(7):1818–22.

Andre C, Andre F, Colin L. Effect of allergen ingestion challenge with and without cromoglycate cover on intestinal permeability in atopic dermatitis, urticaria, and other symptoms of food allergy. Allergy 1989;44(Suppl 9):47–51.

Ankri S, Mirelman D. Antimicrobial properties of allicin from garlic. Microbes Infect 1999;1(2):125–29.

Anton PA. Stress and mind-body impact on the course of inflammatory bowel diseases. Semin Gastrointest Dis 1999;10(1):14–19.

Ball E. Exercise guidelines for patients with inflammatory bowel disease. Gastroenterol Nurs 1998;21(3):108–111.

Barefoot SF, Chen YR, Hughes TA, et al. Identification and purification of a protein that induces production of the Lactobacillus acidophilus bacteriocin lactacin B. Appl Environ Microbiol 1994;60:3522–28.

Barefoot SF, Klaenhammer TR. Detection and activity of lactacin B, a bacteriocin produced by Lactobacillus acidophilus. Appl Environ Microbiol 1983;45:1808–15.

Belluzzi A, Boschi S, Brignola C, Munarini A, Cariani G, Miglio F. Polyunsaturated fatty acids and inflammatory bowel disease. Am J Clin Nutr 2000;71(suppl):339S–342S.

Belluzzi A, Brignola C, Campieri M, et al. Effects of new fish oil derivative on fatty acid phospholipid-membrane pattern in a group of Crohn's disease patients. Dig Dis Sci 1994;39(12):2589–2594.

Belluzzi A, Brignola C, Campieri M, Pera A, Boschi S, Miglioli M. Effect of an enteric-coated fish-oil preparation on relapses in Crohn's disease. N Engl J Med 1996;334(24):1557–1560.

Bensky D, Gamble A. Chinese Herbal Medicine. Seattle: Eastland Press, 1986.

Bernell O, Lapidus A, Hellers G. Risk factors for surgery and postoperative recurrence in Crohn's disease. Ann Surg 2000;231(1):38–45.

Blumenthal M, ed. Herbal Medicine: Expanded Commission E Monographs. Newton, MA: OneMedicine, 2000.

Blumenthal M, Busse WR, Goldberg A, et al., ed. The Complete German Commission E Monographs: Therapeutic Guide to Herbal Medicines. Austin, Texas: American Botanical Society, 1998.

Bock S. Integrative medical treatment of inflammatory bowel disease. Int J Integr Med 2000;2(5):21–29.

Borch E, Rosen C, Bjorck L. Antibacterial effect of the lactoperoxidase/thiocyanate/hydro gen peroxide system against strains of campylobacter isolated from poultry. J Food Protect 1989;42(9):639–41.

Borum ML. Irritable bowel syndrome. Gastroenterology 2001;28(3):523–38.

REFERENCES

Bousvaros A, Zurakowski D, Duggan C. Vitamins A and E serum levels in children and young adults with inflammatory bowel disease: effect of disease activity. J Pediatr Gastroenterol Nutr 1998;26:129–135.

Brignola C, Belloli C, De Simone G, et al. Zinc supplementation restores plasma concentrations of zinc and thymulin in patients with Crohn's disease. Aliment Pharmacol Ther 1993;7:275–280.

Browning SM. Constipation, diarrhea, and irritable bowel syndrome. Prim Care 1999;26(1):113–39.

Cao Y, Feng Z, Hoos A, et al. Glutamine enhances gut glutathione production. J Parent Enteral Nutr 1998;22(4):224–27.

Cassell GH, Mekalanos J. Antibiotic resistance. JAMA 2001;285:601–05.

Chevallier A. The Encyclopedia of Medicinal Plants. London: Dorling Kindersley, 1996.

Chowers Y, Sela B, Holland R, Fidder H, Simoni FB, Bar-Meir S. Increased levels of homocysteine in patients with Crohn's disease are related to folate levels. Am J Gastroenterol 2000;95(12):3498–3502.

Colombel J, Mathieu D, Bouault J, Lesage X, Zavadil P, Quandelle P, Cortot A. Hyperbaric oxygenation in severe perineal Crohn's disease. Dis Colon Rectum 1995;38:609–614.

Conneely OM. Antiinflammatory activities of lactoferrin. J Am Coll Nutr 2001;20(5 Suppl): 389S–97S.

Cosnes J, Beaugerie L, Carbonnel F, Gendre JP. Smoking cessation and the course of Crohn's disease: an intervention study. Gastroenterology 2001;120(5):1093–1099.

Cowan MM. Plant products as antimicrobial agents. Clin Microbiol Rev 1999;12(4):564–82.

Dear KL, Hunter JO. Colonoscopic hydrostatic balloon dilation of Crohn's strictures. J Clin Gastroenterol 2001;33(4):315–318.

Dharmananda S. Chinese Herbology: A Professional Training Program. Portland, Oregon: Institute for Traditional and Preventative Health Care, 1992.

Dorman HJ, Deans SG. Antimicrobial agents from plants: antibacterial activity of plant volatile oils. J Appl Microbiol 2000; 88(2):308–16.

Duke JA. Handbook of Medicinal Herbs. Boca Raton: CRC Press, 1985.

Dunne C. Adaptation of bacteria to the intestinal niche: probiotics and gut disorder. Inflamm Bowel Dis 2001;7(2):136–45.

Duthie SJ, Collins AR, Duthie GG, Dobson VL. Quercetin and myricetin protect against hydrogen peroxide-induced DNA damage (strand breaks and oxidised pyrimidines) in human lymphocytes. Mutat Res. 1997;393(3):223–231.

Ellestad-Sayed J, Nelson R, Adson M, et al. Pantothenic acid, coenzyme A, and human chronic ulcerative and granulomatous colitis. Am J Clin Nutr 1976;29:1333–38.

Ellison RT. The effects of lactoferrin on gram-negative bacteria. Adv Exp Med Biol 1994;357: 71–90.

Entocortä EC (budesonide) for Crohn's disease approved by the FDA. Crohn's and Colitis Foundation of America (October 3, 2001), http://www.ccfa.org/news/entocort.htm (accessed October 15, 2001).

Farmer M, Petras RE, Hunt LE, Janosky JE, Galadiuk S. The importance of diagnostic accuracy in colonic inflammatory bowel disease. Am J Gastroenterol 2000; 95(11): 3184–3188.

Favier C, Neut C, Mizon C, Cortot A, Colombel JF, Mizon J. Fecal ß-D-Galactosidase production and Bifidobacteriaare decreased in Crohn's disease. Dig Dis Sci 1997;42(4): 817–822.

Feagan BG, Fedorak RN, Irvine EJ, et al. A comparison of methotrexate with placebo for the maintenance of remission in Crohn's disease. N Engl J Med 2000;342:1627–1632.

Ferry DR, Smith A, Malkhandi J, et al. Phase I clinical trial of the flavonoid quercetin pharmacokinetics and evidence for in vivo tyrosine kinase inhibition. Clin Cancer Res. 1996;2(4):659–668.

Fleming C, Huizenga K, McCall J, et al. Zinc nutrition in Crohn's disease. Dig Dis Sci 1991;26(10):865–70.

Foster S, Tyler V. Tyler's Honest Herbal. New York: Haworth Press, 1999:97–99.

Fraser AG, Woollard GA. Gastric juice ascorbic acid is related to Helicobacter pylori infection but not ethnicity. J Gastroenterol Hepatol 1999;14(11):1070–73.

Frolov VM, Peresadin NA, Khomutianskaia NI, Pshenichnyi I. The efficacy of quercetin and tocopherol acetate in treating patients with Flexner's dysentery [in Ukrainian]. Lik Sprava 1993;4:84–86.

Galland L, Barrie S. Intestinal dysbiosis and the causes of disease. J Adv Med 1993;6(2):67–81.

Geerling BJ, Badart-Smook A, Stockbrügger RW, Brummer R-JM. Comprehensive nutritional status in recently diagnosed patients with inflammatory bowel disease compared with population controls. Eur J Clin Nutr 2000;54:514–521.

Geerling BJ, Houwelingen AC, Badart-Smook A, Stockbrügger RW, Brummer R-JM. Fat intake and fatty acid profile in plasma phospholipids and adipose tissue in patients with Crohn's disease, compared with controls. Am J Gastroenterol 1999b;94(2):410–417.

Geerling BJ, Houwelingen AC, Badart-Smook A, Stockbrügger RW, Brummer R-JM. The relation between antioxidant status and alterations in fatty acid profile in patients with Crohn disease and controls. Scand J Gastroenterol 1999a;34:1108–1116.

Geerling BJ, Stockbrugger RW, Brummer R-JM. Nutrition and inflammatory bowel disease: an update. Scand J Gastroenterol 1999c;34(suppl 230):95–105.

Genser D, Kang M-H, Vogelsang H, Elmadfa I. Status of lipidsoluble antioxidants and TRAP in patients with Crohn's disease and healthy controls. Eur J Clin Nutr 1999;53:675–679.

Gibson GR, Roberfroid MB. Dietary modulation of the human colonic microbiota: introducing the concept of prebiotics. J Nutr 1995;125:1401–12.

Gill HS, Rutherfurd KJ, Cross ML, et al. Enhancement of immunity in the elderly by dietary supplementation with the probiotic Bifidobacterium lactis HN019. Am J Clin Nutr 2001;74(6):833–39.

Gilliland SE, Nelson CR, Maxwell C. Assimilation of cholesterol by Lactobacillus acidophilus. Appl Environ Microbiol 1985;49:377–81.

Gilliland SE, Speck ML. Antagonistic action of Lactobacillus acidophilus toward intestinal and food borne pathogens in associative cultures. J Food Protection 1977;40(12):820–23.

Gilliland SE, Speck ML, Nauyok DF, et al. Influence of consuming nonfermented milk containing Lactobacillus acidophilus on fecal flora of healthy males. J Dairy Sci 1978;61:1–10.

Gilliland SE, Walker DK. Factors to consider when selecting a culture of Lactobacillus acidophilus as a dietary adjunct to produce a hypocholesterolemic effect in humans. J Dairy Sci 1990;73:905–11.

Gionchetti P, Rizzello F, Venturi A, Campieri M. Probiotics in infective diarrhea and inflammatory bowel diseases. J Gastroenterol Hepatol 2000;15:489–493.

REFERENCES

Gladwin M, Trattler B. Clinical Microbiology Made Ridiculously Simple. Miami: MedMaster, 1995.

Glickman RM. Inflammatory bowel disease: ulcerative colitis and Crohn's disease. In: Fauci AS, Braunwald E, Isselbacher KJ, et al., ed. Harrison's Principles of Internal Medicine, 14th ed. New York: McGraw-Hill, 1998:1633–1645.

Goldin BR, Gorbach SL. Alterations in fecal microflora enzymes related to diet, age, Lactobacillus supplements, and dimethylhydrazine. Cancer 1977;40:2421–26.

Goldin BR, Gorbach SL. Alterations of the intestinal microflora by diet, oral antibiotics, and Lactobacillus: decreased production of free amines from aromatic nitro compounds, azo dyes, and glucuronides. J Natl Cancer Instit 1984;73:689–95.

Goldin BR, Gorbach SL. Effect of Lactobacillus acidophilus dietary supplements on 1,2-dimethylhydrazine dihydrochloride-induced intestinal cancer in rats. J Natl Cancer Instit 1980;64:263–65.

Goldin BR, Gorbach SL. The effect of milk and Lactobacillus feeding on human intestinal bacterial enzyme activity. Amer J Clin Nutr 1984;39:756–61.

Goldin BR, Swenson L, Dwyer J, et al. Effect of diet and Lactobacillus acidophilus supplements on human fecal bacterial enzymes. J Natl Cancer Instit 1980;64:255–61.

Gorbach SL. Estrogens, breast cancer, and intestinal flora. Rev Infect Dis 1984;6(1):S85–S90.

Goto C, Kasuya S, Koga K, et al. Lethal efficacy of extract from Zingiber officinale (traditional Chinese medicine) or [6]-shogaol and [6]-gingerol in Anisakis larvae in vitro. Parisitol Res 1990;76:653–56.

Greene JD, Klaenhammer TR. Factors involved in adherence of lactobacilli to human caco-2 cells. Appl Environ Microbiol 1994;60:4487–94.

Gross M, Pfeiffer M, Martini M, Campbell D, Slavin J, Potter J. The quantitation of metabolites of quercetin flavonols in human urine. Cancer Epidemiol Biomarkers Prevent 1996;5(9):711–720.

Gupta I, Parihar A, Malhotra P, Singh GB, Ludtke R, Safayhi H, Ammon HPT. Effects of Boswellia serrata gum resin in patients with ulcerative colitis. Eur J Med Res 1997;2:37–43.

Guyton AC. Protein Metabolism. In: Textbook of Medical Physiology, 8th ed. Philadelphia: W.B. Saunders, 1991.

Haas EM. Staying Healthy with Nutrition. Berkley, Calif: Celestial Arts Publishing, 1992:272, 882–884.

Haas I, McClain C, Varilek G. Complementary and alternative medicine and gastrointestinal diseases. Curr Opin Gastroenterol 2000;16:188–196.

Hagmar B, Ryd W, Skomedal H. Arabinogalactan blockade of experimental metastases to liver by murine hepatoma. Invasion Metastasis 1991;11(6):348–55.

Hammer KA, Carson CF, Riley TV. Antimicrobial activity of essential oils and other plant extracts. J Appl Microbiol 1999;86(6):985–90.

Hampe J, Cuthbert A, Croucher JP, et al. Association between insertion mutation in NOD2 gene Crohn's disease in German and British populations. Lancet 2001; 357:1925–1928.

Hauer J, Anderer FE. Mechanism of stimulation of human natural killer cytotoxicity by a rabinogalactan from Larix occidentalis. Cancer Immunol Immunother 1993;36(4):237–44.

Hendricks K, Walder W. Zinc deficiency in inflammatory bowel disease. Nutr Rev 1988;46(12):401–08.

Heumann D, Glauser MP. Pathogenesis of sepsis. Sci Am 1994;1:28–37.

REFERENCES

Heuschkel RB, Menache CC, Megerian JT, Baird AE. Enteral nutrition and corticosteroids in the treatment of acute Crohn's disease in children. J Pediatr Gastroenterol Nutr 2000;31(1):8–15.

Hills JM, Aaronson PI. The mechanism of action of peppermint oil on gastro-intestinal smooth muscle. An analysis using patch clamp electrophysiology and isolated tissue pharmacology in rabbit and guinea pig. Gastroenterology 1991;101(1):55–65.

Hollman PC, Van Trijp JM, Mengelers MJ, De Vries JH, Katan, MB. Bioavailability of the dietary antioxidant flavonol quercetin in man. Cancer Lett 1997;114(1–2):139–140.

Horwittz BJ, Fisher RS. The irritable bowel syndrome. New Engl J Med 2001;344(24):1846–50.

Hoyos AB. Reduced incidence of necrotizing enterocolitis associated with enteral administration of Lactobacillus acidophilus and Bifidobacterium infantis to neonates in an intensive care unit. Int J Infect Dis 1999;3(4):197–202.

Huang KC. The Pharmacology of Chinese Herbs. Boca Raton: CRC Press, 1993.

Irritable bowel syndrome. National Institutes of Health, National Institute of Diabetes and Digestive and Kidney Diseases (October 1992), http://www.niddk.nih.gov/health/digest/pubs/irrbowel/irrbowel.htm (accessed February 5, 2002).

Isolauri E, Juntunen M, Wiren S. Intestinal permeability changed in acute gastroenteritis: effects of clinical factors and nutritional management. J Pediatr Gastroenterol Nutr 1989;8(4):466–73.

Janowitz HD, Croen EC, Sacher DB. The role of the fecal stream in Crohn's disease: an historical and analytical review. Inflamm Bowel Dis 1998;4(1):29–39.

Joachim G. The relationship between habits of food consumption and reported reactions to food in people with inflammatory bowel disease—testing the limits. Nutr Health 1999;13(2):69–83.

Johnson HM, Torres BA, Soos JM. Superantigens:structure and relevance to human disease. Soc Exp Biol Med 1996;212:99–109.

Jonas WB, Jacobs J. Healing with Homeopathy: The Doctors' Guide. New York: Warner, 1996: 220.

Kaneda Y, Torii M, Tanaka T, et al. In vitro effects of berberine sulphate on the growth and structure of Entamoeba histolytica, Giardia lamblia and Trichomonas vaginalis. Annals Trop Med Parasitology 1991;85(4):417–25.

Kaplan H, Hutkins RW. Fermentation of fructooligosaccharides by lactic acid bacteria and bifidobacteria. Appl Environ Microbiol 2000;66(6):2682–84.

Keane J, Gershon S, Wise RP, et al. Tuberculosis associated with infliximab, a tumor necrosis factor alpha-neutralizing agent. N Engl J Med 2001;345(15):1098–1104.

Kelly GS. Larch arabinogalactan: clinical relevance of a novel immune-enhancing polysaccharide. Alt Med Rev. 1999;4(2):96–103.

Kim GS, Gilliland SE. Lactobacillus acidophilus as a dietary adjunct for milk to aid lactose digestion in humans. J Dairy Sci 1983;66:959–66.

Klaenhammer TR. Microbiological considerations in selection and preparation of Lactobacillus strains for use as dietary adjuncts. J Dairy Sci 1982;65:1339–49.

Klaenhammer TR, Kleeman EG. Growth characteristics, bile sensitivity, and freeze damage in colonial variants of Lactobacillus acidophilus. Appl Environ Microbiol 1981;41:1461–67.

Kleeman EG, Klaenhammer TR. Adherence of Lactobacillus species to human fetal intestinal cells. J Dairy Sci 1982;65:2063–69.

Klimberg VS, Salloum RM, Kasper M, et al. Oral glutamine accelerates healing of the small intestine and improves outcome after whole abdominal radiation. Arch Surg 1990;125(8):1040–45.

REFERENCES

Kline RM, Kline JJ, Di Palma J, et al. Enteric-coated, pH-dependent peppermint oil capsules for the treatment of irritable bowel syndrome in children. J Pedriatr 2001;138(1):125–28.

Knekt P, Jarvinen R, Reunanen A, Maatela J. Flavonoid intake and coronary mortality in Finland: a cohort study. BMJ (Clinical Research Ed) 1996;312(7029):478–481.

Knoke M, Bernhardt H. The impact of microbial ecology on clinical problems. Infection 1989;17(4):255–58.

Koch HP, Lawson LD, ed. Garlic: The Science and Therapeutic Application of Allium sativum L. and Related Species, 2nd ed. Baltimore: Williams and Wilkins, 1996.

Kruzel ML, Harari Y, Chen C-Y, et al. The gut: a key metabolic organ protected by lactoferrin during experimental systemic inflammation in mice. Adv Exp Med Biol 1998;443:167–73.

Kucera LS, Cohen RA, Herrmann EC. Antiviral activities of extracts of the lemon balm plant. Ann NY Acad Sci 1965;130(1):474–82.

Kurinets A, Lichtenberger LM. Phosphatidylcholine-associated aspirin accelerates healing of gastric ulcers in rats. Dig Dis Sci 1998;43(4):786–90.

Kuroki F, Iida M, Matsumoto T, Aoyagi K, Kanamoto K, Fujishima M. Serum n3 polyunsatu rated fatty acids are depleted in Crohn's disease. Dig Dis Sci 1997;42(6):1137–1141.

Kuroki F, Iida M, Tominaga M, et al. Multiple vitamin status in Crohn's disease. Dig Dis Sci 1993;38(9):1614–1618.

Kussendrager KD, van Hooijdonk AC. Lactoperoxidase: physico-chemical properties, occurrence, mechanism of action and applications. Br J Nutr 2000;84 (Suppl 1):S19–25.

Lacroix B, Didier E, Grenier J. Role of pantothenic and ascorbic acid in wound healing processes: in vitro study on fibroblasts. Intl J Vit Nutr Res 1988;58:507–13.

Lavy A, Weisz G, Adir Y, Ramon Y, Melamed Y, Eidelman S. Hyperbaric oxygen for perianal Crohn's disease. J Clin Gastroenterol 1994;19(3):202–205.

LeLeiko NS, Walsh MJ. The role of glutamine, short-chain fatty acids, and nucleotides in intestinal adaptation to gastrointestinal disease. Pediatr Clin North Am 1996;43(2):451–70.

Lengerich EJ, Addiss DG. Severe giardiasis in the United States. Clin Infec Dis 1994; 18:760–63.

Levy E, Rizwan Y, Thibault L, et al. Altered lipid profile, lipoprotein composition, and oxidant and antioxidant status in pediatric Crohn disease. Am J Clin Nutr 2000;71:807–815.

Levy SB. The challenge of antibiotic resistance. Sci Am 1998;278(3):46–53.

Lewis DA, Shaw GP. A natural flavonoid and synthetic analogues protect the gastric mucosa from aspirin-induced erosions. J Nutr Biochem 2001;12(2):85–100.

Lewis JD, Fisher RL. Nutrition support in inflammatory bowel disease. Med Clin North Am 1994;78(6):1443–1456.

Lih-Brody L, Powell SR, Collier KP, et al. Increased oxidative stress and decreased antioxidant defenses in mucosa of inflammatory bowel disease. Dig Dis Sci 1996;41(10):2078–2086.

Lin MY, Savaiano D, Harlander S. Influence of nonfermented dairy products containing bacterial starter cultures on lactose maldigestion in humans. J Dairy Sci 1991;74:87–95.

Lis-Balchin M, Hart S. Studies on the mode of action of the essential oil of lavender (Lavandula angustifolia P. Miller). Phytother Res 1999;13(6):540–42.

Liu JH, Chen GH, Yeh HZ, et al. Enteric-coated peppermint oil capsules in the treatment of irritable bowel syndrome: a prospective, randomized trial. J Gastroenterol 1997;32(6):765–68.

REFERENCES

Loudon CP, Corroll V, Butcher J, Rawsthorne P, Bernstein CN. The effects of physical exercise on patients with Crohn's disease. Am J Gastroenterol 1999;94(3):697–703.

Malin M, Suomalainen H, Saxelin M, Isolauri E. Promotion of IgA immune response in patients with Crohn's disease by oral bacteriotherapy with LactobacillusGG. Ann Nutr Metab 1996;40:137–145.

Marteau PR, de Vrese M, Cellier CJ, et al. Protection from gastrointestinal diseases with the use of probiotics. Am J Clin Nutr 2001;73(suppl):430S–36S.

Mascolo N, Jain R, Jain SC, et al. Ethnopharmacologic investigation of ginger (Zingiber officinale). J Ethnopharmacol 1989;27:129–40.

Mayer EA. Emerging disease model for functional gastrointestinal disorders. Am J Med 1999;107(5A):12S–19S.

McCarthy DM. Comparative toxicity of nonsteroidal anti-inflammatory drugs. Am J Med 1999;107(6A):37S–46S.

McDowell RM, McElvaine MD. Long-term sequelae of foodborne diseases. Rev Sci Tech 1997;16(2):337–41.

Mielants H, De Vos M, Goemaere S, et al. Intestinal mucosal permeability in inflammatory rheumatic diseases. II. Role of disease. J Rheumatol 1991;18(3):394–400.

Milhau G, Valentin A, Benoit F, et al. In vitro antimalarial activity of eight essential oils. J Essent Oil Res 1997;9:329–33.

Montes RG, Bayless TM, Saavedra JM. Effect of milks inoculated with Lactobacillus acidophilus or a yogurt starter culture in lactose-maldigesting children. J Dairy Sci 1995;78(8):1657–64.

Msika S, Iannelli A, Deroide G, et al. Can laparoscopy reduce hospital stay in the treatment of Crohn's disease? Dis Colon Rectum 2001;44(11):1661–1666.

Mukhopadhyaya K, Bhattacharya D, Chakraborty A, et al. Effect of banana powder (Musa sapeintus var. paradisiaca) on gastric mucosal shedding. J Ethnopharmacol 1987; 21(1):11–19.

Mulder TPJ, Van Der Sluys Veer A, Verspaget HW, et al. Effect of oral zinc supplementation on metallothionein and superoxide dismutase concentrations in patients with inflammatory bowel disease. J Gastroenterol Hepatol 1994;9:472–477.

Munkholm P, Langholz E, Hollander D, et al. Intestinal permeability in patients with Crohn's disease and ulcerative colitis and their first degree relatives. Gut 1994;35(1):68–72.

Murray MT. Encyclopedia of Nutritional Supplements. Rocklin, Calif: Prima, 1996: 320–321.

Murray MT, Pizzorno JE. Encyclopedia of Natural Medicine, 2nd ed. Rocklin, Calif: Prima, 1996:268, 314, 422, 494, 546–47, 766.

Nakajima M, Shinoda I, Samejima Y, et al. Lactoferrin as a suppressor of cell migration of gastrointestinal cell lines. J Cell Physiol 1997;170(2):101–05.

Niebauer J, Volk HD, Kemp M, et al. Endotoxin and immune activation in chronic heart failure: a prospective cohort study. Lancet 1999;353(9167):1838–42.

Noyer CM, Brandt LJ. Hyperbaric oxygen therapy for perineal Crohn's disease. Am J Gastroenterol 1999;94(2):318–321.

O'Hara MA, Kiefer D, Farrell K, et al. A review of 12 commonly used medicinal herbs. Arch Fam Med 1998;7(6):523–36.

Olaison G, Sjodahl R, Tagesson C. Abnormal intestinal permeability in Crohn's disease. Scand J Gastroenterol 1990;25(4):321–28.

Pearson M, Teahon K, Levi AJ, Bjarnason I. Food intolerance and Crohn's disease. Gut 1993;34:783–787.

REFERENCES

Philipsen-Geerling BJ, Brummer RJM. Nutrition in Crohn's disease. Curr Opin Clin Nutr Metab Care 2000;3:305–309.

Rabbani GH, Butler T, Knight J, et al. Randomized controlled trial of berberine sulfate therapy for diarrhea due to enterotoxigenic Eschericia coli and Vibrio cholerae. J Infec Dis 1987;155(5):979–84.

Rajapakse R, Korelitz BI. Inflammatory bowel disease during pregnancy. Current Treatment Options in Gastroenterology 2001;4(3):245–251.

Rannem T, Ladefoged K, Hylander E, Hegnhøj J, Staun M. Selenium depletion in patients with gastrointestinal diseases: are there any predictive factors? Scand J Gastroenterol 1998;33:1057–1061.

Rasic JLJ, Kurmann JA. Bifidobacteria and Their Role. Boston: Kirkhauser Verlag, 1983.

Rawsthorne P, Shanahan F, Cronin NC, et al. An international survey of the use and attitudes regarding alternative medicine by patients with inflammatory bowel disease. Am J Gastroenterol 1999;94(5):1298–1303.

Reed PI. Vitamin C, Helicobacter pylori infection and gastric carcinogenesis. Int J Vitam Nutr Res 1999;69(3):220–27.

Reid G. In vitro testing of Lactobacillus acidophilus NCFM as a possible probiotic for the urogenital tract. Int Dairy J 2000;10:415–19.

Reid G. The scientific basis for probiotic strains of Lactobacillus. Appl Environ Microbiol 1999;65(9):3763–66.

Remicade (infliximab)–black box warning. U.S. Food and Drug Administration (FDA) Med Watch (October 23, 2001), http://www.fda.gov/medwatch/SAFETY/2001/safety01.htm (accessed October 23, 2001).

Research on host susceptibility to emerging pathogens. National Institutes of Health, National Institute of Allergy and Infectious Disease (n.d.), http://www.niaid.nih.gov/publications/execsum/3a.htm (accessed April 3, 2000).

Rhee JK, Woo KJ, Baek BK, et al. Screening of the wormicidal Chinese raw drugs on Clonorchis sinensis. Am J Chin Med 1982;9(4):277–84.

Ringel Y, Drossman DA. Psychosocial aspects of Crohn's disease. Surg Clin North Am 2001;81(1):231–252.

Ringel Y, Sperber AD, Drossman DA. Irritable bowel syndrome. Annu Rev Med 2001; 52:319–38.

Rioux JD, Daly MJ, Silverberg MS, et al. Genetic variation in the 5q31 cytokine gene cluster confers susceptibility to Crohn disease. Nat Genet 2001;29:223–228.

Roberfroid MB. Chicory fructooligosaccharides and the gastrointestinal tract. Nutrition 2000;16(7–8):677–79.

Robinson R, Causey J, Slavin JL. Nutritional benefits of larch arabinogalactan. In: McCleary BV, Prosky L, ed. Advanced Dietary Fibre Technology. London: Blackwell Science 2001: 443–51.

Rowlands BJ, Gardiner KR. Nutritional modulation of gut inflammation. Proc Nutr Soc 1998;57(3):395–401.

Russel MG. Changes in the incidence of inflammatory bowel disease: what does it mean? Eur J Intern Med 2000;11(4):191–196.

Salvatore S, Heuschkel R, Tomlin S, et al. A pilot study of N-acetyl glucosamine, a nutritional substrate for glycosaminoglycan synthesis, in pediatric chronic inflammatory bowel disease. Aliment Pharmacol Ther 2000;14:1567–1579.

Samartín S, Marcos A, Chandra RK. Food hypersensitivity. Nutr Res 2001;21(3):473–97.

REFERENCES

Sanders ME, Klaenhammer TR. The scientific basis of Lactobacillus acidophilus NCFM functionality as a probiotic. J Dairy Sci 2001;84:319–31.

Sanders ME, Walker DC, Walker KM, et al. Performance of commercial cultures in fluid milk applications. J Dairy Sci 1996;79:943–55.

Schauss AG. Lactobacillus acidophilus: method of action, clinical application, and toxicity data. J Adv Med 1990;3(3):163–78.

Schulz V, Hansel R, Tyler VE. Rational Phytotherapy: A Physicians' Guide to Herbal Medicine, 3rd ed. Berlin: Springer-Verlag, 1998.

Schuster MM. Defining and diagnosing irritable bowel syndrome. Amer J Man Care 2001;7(Suppl):S247–51.

Shanahan F. Probiotics and inflammatory bowel disease: is there a scientific rationale? Inflamm Bowel Dis 2000;6(2):107–115.

Shils ME, Olson JA, Shike M, et al., ed. Modern Nutrition in Health and Disease, 9th ed. Baltimore: Williams and Wilkins, 1999.

Shils ME, Olson JA, Shike M, Ross AC. Modern Nutrition in Health and Disease, 9th ed. Baltimore: Williams and Wilkins; 1999:1274–1277.

Shin K, Hayasawa H, Lonnerdal B. Inhibition of Escherichia coli respiratory enzymes by the lactoperoxidase-hydrogen peroxide-thiocyanate antimicrobial system. J Appl Microbiol 2001;90(4):489–93.

Shin K, Yamauchi K, Teraguchi S, et al. Susceptibility of Helicobacter pylori and its urease activity to the peroxidase-hydrogen peroxide-thiocyanate antimicrobial system. J Med Microbiol 2002;51(3):231–37.

Sicherer SH. Manifestations of food allergy: evaluation and management. Am Fam Physician 1999; 59(2):415–24, 429–30.

Sicherer SH, Sampson HA. Food hypersensitivity and atopic dermatitis: pathophysiology, epidemiology, diagnosis, and management. J Allergy Clin Immunol 1999;104(3 Pt 2): S114–22.

Simenhoff ML, Dunn SR, Zollner GP, et al. Biomodulation of the toxic and nutritional effects of small bowel bacterial overgrowth in end-stage kidney disease using freeze-dried Lactobacillus acidophilus. Miner Electrolyte Metab 1996;22:92–96.

Skov L, Baadsgaard O. Superantigens: do they have a role in skin disease? Arch Dermatol 1995;131(7):829–32.

Slocum MM, Sittig MD, Specian RD, et al. Absence of intestinal bile promotes bacterial translocation. Am Surg 1992;58:305–10.

Slonim AE, Bulone L, Damore MB, Goldberg T, Wingertzahn MA, McKinley MJ. A preliminary study of growth hormone therapy for Crohn's disease. N Engl J Med 2000;342:1633–1637.

Smith M, Gibson R, Brooks P. Abnormal bowel permeability in ankylosing spondylitis and rheumatoid arthritis. J Rheumatol 1985;12(2):299–305.

Smith-Palmer A, Stewart J, Fyfe L. Antimicrobial properties of plant essential oils and essences against five important food-borne pathogens. Lett Appl Microbiol 1998;26(2):118–22.

Soos JM, Schiffenbauer J, Torres BA, et al. Superantigens as virulence factors in autoimmunity and immunodeficiency diseases. Med Hypotheses 1997;48(3):253–59.

Souba WW, Klimberg VS, Plumley DA, et al. The role of glutamine in maintaining a healthy gut and supporting the metabolic response to injury and infection. J Surgical Res 1990;48(4):383–91.

Steger GG, Mader RM, Vogelsang H, Schöfl R, Lochs H, Ferenci P. Folate absorption in Crohn's disease. Digestion 1994;55:234–238.

REFERENCES

Stein RB, Lichtenstein GR, Rombeau JL. Nutrition in inflammatory bowel disease. Curr Opin Clin Nutr Metab Care 1999;2:367–371.

Sy ND, Hoan DB, Dung NP, et al. Treatment of malaria in Vietnam with oral artemisinin. Am J Trop Med Hyg 1993;48(3):398–402.

Szulc P, Meunier PJ. Is vitamin K deficiency a risk factor for osteoporosis in Crohn's disease? [commentary]. Lancet 2001;357(9273):1995–1996.

Tabak M, Armon R, Potaman I, et al. In vitro inhibition of Helicobacter pylori by extracts of thyme. J Appl Bacteriol 1996;80(6):667–72.

Takeshima F, Makiyama K, Doi T. Hyperbaric Oxygen as adjunct therapy for Crohn's intractable enteric ulcer. Am J Gastroenterol 1999;94(11):3374–3375.

Talal AH, Drossman DA. Psychosocial factors in inflammatory bowel disease. Gastroenterol Clin North Am 1995;24(3):699–716.

Teahon K, Bjarnason I, Pearson M, Levi AJ. Ten years' experience with an elemental diet in the management of Crohn's disease. Gut 1990;31(10):1133–1137.

Thomas EL, Milligan TW, Joyner RE, et al. Antibacterial activity of hydrogen peroxide and the lactoperoxidase-hydrogen peroxide-thiocyanate system against oral streptococci. Infect Imm 1994;6(2):529–35.

Tomomatsu H. Health effects of oligosaccharides. Food Tech 1994;October:61–65.

Torres BA, Johnson HM. Modulation of disease by superantigens. Curr Opin Immunol 1998;10(4):465–70.

Tsujikawa T, Satoh J, Katsuhiro U, et al. Clinical importance of n-3 fatty acid-rich diet and nutritional education for the maintenance of remission in Crohn's disease. Gastroenterol 2000;35:99–104.

Tuomola E, Crittenden R, Playne M, et al. Quality assurance criteria for probiotic bacteria. Am J Clin Nutr 2001;73(suppl):393S–98S.

Tyler VE, Brady LR, Robbers, JE. Pharmacognosy, 9th ed. Philadelphia: Lea and Febiger, 1988.

Ullman D. The Consumer's Guide to Homeopathy.New York: Penguin Putnam, 1995: 76–77.

Ullman D. Homeopathic Medicine for Children and Infants. New York: Penguin Putnam, 1992: 244–245.

United States Food and Drug Administration (FDA). FDA approves new treatment for Crohn's disease. FDA Talk Paper. October 3, 2001. Number T01–45.

Van der Strate BW, Beljaars L, Molema G, et al. Antiviral activities of lactoferrin. Antiviral Res 2001;52(3):225–39.

Van Heel DA, McGovern DPB, Jewell DP. Crohn's disease: a genetic susceptibility, bacteria, and innate immunity [commentary]. Lancet 2001;357:1902–1903.

Van Hooijdonk AC, Kussendrager KD, Steijns JM. In vivo antimicrobial and antiviral activity of components in bovine milk and colostrum involved in non-specific defence. Br J Nutr 2000;84(Suppl 1):S127–34.

Veys EM, Mielants H. Enteropathic arthritis, uveitis, Whipple's disease, and miscellaneous spondyloarthropathies. Curr Opin Rheumatol 1993;5(4):420–27.

Vince AJ, McNeil NI, Wager JD, et al. The effect of lactulose, pectin, arabinogalactan and cellulose on the production of organic acids and metabolism of ammonia by intestinal bacteria in a faecal incubation system. Br J Nutr 1990;63(1):17–26.

Vogelsang H, Ferenci P, Resch H, Kiss A, Gangl A. Prevention of bone mineral loss in patients with Crohn's disease by long-term oral vitamin D supplementation. Eur J Gastroenterol Hepatol 1995;7:609–614.

REFERENCES

Wakabayashi H, Orihara T, Nakaya A, et al. Effect of Helicobacter pylori infection on gastric mucosal phospholipid contents and their fatty acid composition. J Gastrenterol Hepatol 1998;13(6):566–71.

Walker DK, Gilliland SE. Relationships among bile tolerance, bile salt deconjugation, and assimilation of cholesterol by Lactobacillus acidophilus. J Dairy Sci 1993;76:956–61.

Wallace JM. Nutritional modulation of gut-immune system interactions in autoimmunity. Int J Integr Med 2000;2(1):18–22.

Wang M, Shao Y, Li J, et al. Antioxidative phenolic glycosides from sage (Salvia officinalis). J Nat Prod 1999;62(3):454–56.

Ward PP, Uribe-Luna S, Conneely OM. Lactoferrin and host defense. Biochem Cell Biol 2002;80(1):95–102.

Werbach MR. Nutritional Influences on Illness, 2nd ed. Tarzana, Calif: Third Line Press, 1993:179, 259, 267, 389.

Wollowski I, Rechkemmer G, Pool-Zobel BL. Protective role of probiotics and prebiotics in colon cancer. Am J Clin Nutr 2001;73(suppl):451S–55S.

Yamahara J, Huang Q, Li Y, et al. Gastrointestinal motility enhancing effect of ginger and its active constituents. Chem Pharm Bull 1990;38(2):430–31.

Young JF, Nielsen SE, Haraldsdottir J, et al. Effect of fruit juice intake on urinary quercetin excretion and biomarkers of antioxidative status. Am J Clin Nutr 1999; 69(1):87–94.

Zachos M, Tondeur M, Griffiths AM. Enteral nutritional therapy for inducing remission of Crohn's disease (Cocrane Review). In: The Cochrane Library, 4, 2001. Oxford: Update Software.

Ziegler TR, Bazargan N, Leader LM, et al. Glutamine and the gastrointestinal tract. Curr Opin Clin Nutr Metab Care 2000;3(5):355–62.

Zurita VF, Rawls DE, Dyck WP. Nutritional support in inflammatory bowel disease. Dig Dis 1995;13:92–107.